the first forty days

The Essential Art of
Nourishing the New Mother

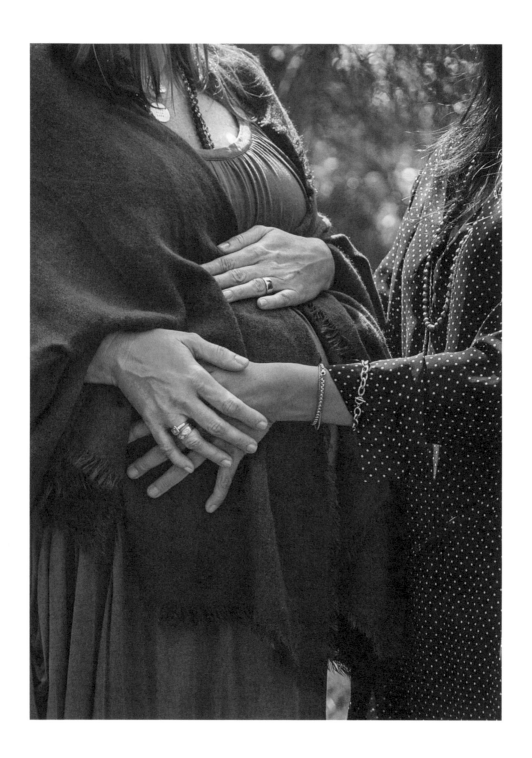

the first forty days

The Essential Art of Nourishing the New Mother

HENG OU

WITH AMELY GREEVEN AND MARISA BELGER
PHOTOGRAPHS BY JENNY NELSON

Abrams | New York

Published in 2016 by Abrams

Library of Congress Control Number: 2015948994

ISBN: 978-1-61769-183-6

EDITOR: Holly Dolce
DESIGNER: Laura Palese
PRODUCTION MANAGER: Anet Sirna-Bruder
PHOTOGRAPHER: Jenny Nelson
FOOD STYLIST: Nicole Kruzick

Printed and bound in the U.S.A.

10 9 8 7

Abrams books are available at special discounts when
purchased in quantity for premiums and promotions as well as fundraising
or educational use. Special editions can also be created to specification. For details,
contact specialsales@abramsbooks.com or the address below.

None of what follows is intended to replace the care and advice offered
by your physician or health-care provider. Please use the food and advice in
The First Forty Days to enhance and improve your day-to-day experience, not to remedy actual
medical issues. However, should you experience any unusual or uncomfortable
symptoms before or after the baby arrives that aren't resolved by your health-care provider,
use this book as a launching pad toward an experienced Chinese medicine doctor.
He or she may be able to offer you herbs and treatment that can be extremely effective in
supporting your body to heal and find its balance for the future.

ABRAMS The Art of Books
195 Broadway, New York, NY 10007
abramsbooks.com

WITH GRATITUDE...

To my children Khefri, India, and Jude; and to their father who helped me create these three bright stars.

To my courageous writers Amely Greeven and Marisa Belger, who, inspired by the challenges of their own postpartum experiences, took on this project with me, determined to create a guidepost for all the mothers who will come after them; and to my agent, Marc Gerald, the connector who brought us together. Without this dynamic literary trio, this book would not have been seen by Holly Dolce, Rebecca Kaplan, and the rest of the fabulous Abrams team.

Big thanks and love to all the experts who shared their wisdom and the beautiful mothers who invited us into their first forty days, giving us a peek into daily life with their new babies. Thank you Jenny Nelson, for your unique photographic perspective and invaluable organizational skills; Nicole Kruzick, for the luscious food styling; and to all of the guides and friends who make up my family: Linda Costigan, Ani Compton, Jessica Janney, Stacy Sindlinger, Toni Spencer, Ian Scanlan, Joe Sturges, Rob Lam, Davi Khalsa, James Ballard, Hsuan Ou, my mama, and the MotherBees team.

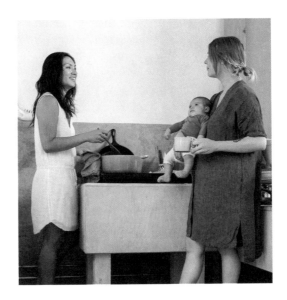

contents

INTRODUCTION

The first forty days is a period of time unlike any other. It is a short season of life that follows the delivery of your child—an almost six-week-long period that arrives after many weeks of pregnancy and who knows how many hours of labor—in which you recover from birth, your baby unfurls slowly into the world of bright lights and sounds, and together you devote yourselves to forging your relationship outside the womb.

Though brief, it is a time of amazing intensity and massive adjustment.

Your body transforms—again—and your heart throbs with more feelings than you ever knew possible. Your internal rhythms ping-pong as days and nights merge. Your stamina and serenity get tested like never before. Your connections to the world you knew before loosen, or even come undone, and your sense of who you are begins to change and morph.

In other times, and in other places around the world, a postpartum period of healing and adjustment was expected and allowed. After the rigorous and demanding act of birth, it was considered critically necessary for the whole family—and for society at large—that a woman be given the first forty days to heal and rest. Other people in her community would feed her, nurture her, and take all responsibilities off her plate, so that she could focus on one thing only: transitioning healthily and happily from expectant woman to mother.

For the first forty days—or sometimes the first thirty or twenty-one, depending on the culture—a new mother stayed secluded from the busy stream of life, tucked indoors with her infant at her side. She received special meals to rebuild energy, replenish lost nutrients, and help her body produce breast milk. She followed traditional practices of keeping rested and warm to prevent exhaustion and depletion.

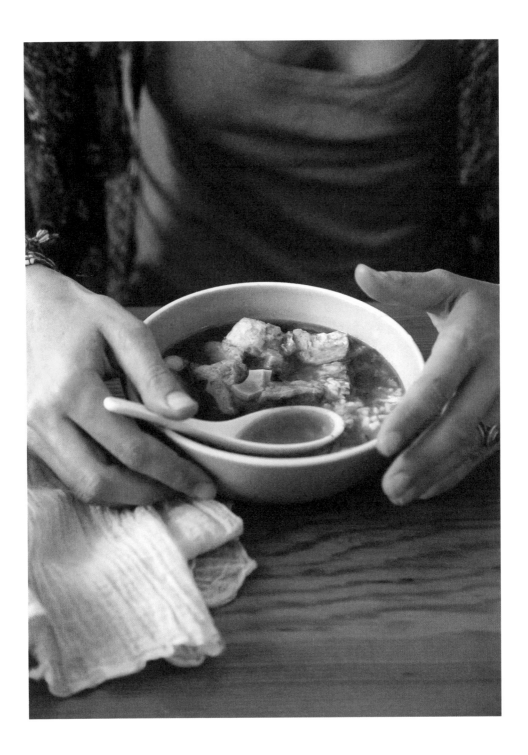

The understanding was that the new mother was as vulnerable as her newborn, requiring her own steady stream of attention and care. A dedicated time of postpartum recovery could help to keep future illness—and equally important, depression—at bay.

Today in the West, we are waking up to the importance of cocooning baby in the weeks following birth. The understanding that he (or she) is not quite ready to meet the world-at-large when he emerges and is still in an early stage of development that's come to be known as the "fourth trimester" has awakened us to the value of holding him close and sheltered for some weeks, so he can shift slowly and gradually into life outside the womb.

But somehow, we have forgotten the time-honored wisdom that this special cocoon of care should extend to the mother as well. In those first forty days, which roughly correlate with the six-week phase that Western medicine calls the postpartum period, the old ways teach that an amazing opportunity presents itself to a woman. During this time, she can revitalize herself and replenish her reserves, creating a solid foundation from which to tackle the demands of mothering (whether for the first time, the second, or more). Furthermore, they teach that with the right postpartum care, a mother can preserve her reproductive health for future children or eventually experience an easy menopause, aging gracefully over the decades to come.

Perhaps because pregnancy and birth get all the magazine covers and headlines—no surprise, as these events sell more stuff—we've overlooked this last part of the childbearing story. A woman's postpartum experience might be given a brief nod at the end of a pregnancy book, or thirty seconds of footage at the end of a TV show, but a deeper look almost never occurs. Rather than get invited to take a sacred time-out after delivering her child, the new mother is more likely met with pressure to "bounce back"—back to her pre-pregnancy productivity, back to her pre-pregnancy body, and back to her pre-pregnancy spirits.

But when it comes to becoming a mother, there is no back; there is only through. After birthing her child, every woman must pass through this initial adjustment phase. It is a strange and beautiful limbo zone that is both exhausting and exciting, mysterious and monotonous. When she arrives at the other side of the postpartum phase after roughly a month and a half, she will most certainly be facing forward, prepared to take her next steps into motherhood.

The First Forty Days is a gentle guide to this transformative time. Its simple plan of nourishment and support is inspired by the global traditions of maternal care that have existed for millennia. It shares simple wisdom about the healing foods to eat, the teas and herbs to drink, and the small steps you can take to prepare for postpartum. But it is a new guide for a new era, intended to help a modern mother move through her first weeks of motherhood with gusto and grace.

It was born of my own postpartum experience as the American-born descendant of a line of Chinese healers. My relatives inducted me into the Chinese tradition of postpartum care known as *zuo yuezi*, and the experience led me to create a business devoted to feeding mothers the nourishing foods they need to thrive after birth. Having fed scores of moms in the days and weeks following their deliveries, I've become convinced that nutrient-rich postpartum meals, served along with a hearty dose of TLC, play a pivotal role in supporting mom's physical recovery and her mental state, helping to instill in her confidence and calm.

The book includes my favorite postpartum recipes for healing soups, replenishing meals and snacks, and warming, calming, lactation-boosting teas. The recipes are rooted in traditional ways of cooking and use a few specialty ingredients, but the emphasis is on simplicity. The nurturing and therapeutic dishes feature easy-to-source staple foods, appealing handfuls of fresh produce, and effortless cooking techniques that fit the way we use our kitchens today. And these foods can be put together by almost anyone, so that mom and her partner can get on with the good stuff—learning everything there is to know about their beloved child.

I've also had a front-row view of what is sorely lacking in our contemporary culture—a dedicated space and time that allows a woman to "become" a mother at her own pace. It's hard to reconcile the unique needs of postpartum with the demands of our fast-paced, highly productive society—how can we slow down and do less in a world that's continually asking us to do more? All too often, women experience a stressful clash of the two. For many mothers, the joy of a baby's arrival is mixed up with harder feelings: isolation and loneliness after the initial welcoming buzz subsides; bewildering fatigue from trying to hold it all together, or confusion and shame when they cannot.

To help bring balance back into this conundrum, *The First Forty Days* tucks its recommendations for healing foods inside a broader universe of care. I'll share some advice on asking for and arranging a system of help during your postpartum period, creating an optimal environment for restoration and breastfeeding, preparing your relationship for the changes to come, and tending kindly to your body and mind with small acts of self-care. You'll also find insights and words of inspiration from some wise women—and a couple of men—who have hundreds of years of postpartum experience among them. These are this book's version of a circle of elders—something that used to be a presence in every village or community—and they will be there for you should you need them on a long or lonely night, or in the trying moments when the magic of mothering slips into the mundane (as it will definitely do). *The First Forty Days* is much more than a cookbook; it is a field guide to making the most of this wonderfully unpredictable phase of life. It exists to put the spotlight of attention and care on the mother—the very person whose needs can sometimes get lost in the excitement of a new baby.

Just as traditional ways brought a circle of women together to care for a new mother, *The First Forty Days* is also a collective effort. When I had the idea for this book, I reached out to a writer friend, Amely Greeven, to help bring my thoughts to life. She, in turn, brought in another writer and friend, Marisa Belger, to collaborate on wordsmithing the project. Between the three of us, we were mothering six children as we wrote *The First Forty Days*, ranging in ages from under one to eleven years old. We had unique postpartum experiences, yet were united by a clear vision and goal: to empower women to seek the care and nurturing they deserve after bringing a baby into the world. A fourth friend, recipe developer and photographer Jenny Nelson, joined our village to lovingly cook and test each recipe, ensuring that the food and drinks were as simple to make as I'd intended, and beautiful to look at, too. Writing late at night and between nap times and school runs, and cooking vats of bone broths and hearty stews alongside kids' breakfasts, we captured and recorded the information in this book. Throughout the process, we kept one another inspired and uplifted with honest stories from our own first weeks with our babies. We examined and reexamined what would have made that fundamental period better, easier, and sweeter, and then put the answers in this book. My hope is that you, too, will feel our presences beside you, and know that by committing to give yourself the first forty days to heal and adjust to being a mom (at any level and in any way), you are connecting to a web of women who truly have walked in your shoes.

The First Forty Days is not a medical book about pregnancy, birth, and postpartum. There are plenty of those. It will not tell you everything about "what to expect." Instead, it is an invitation to lay the groundwork for a healthy and happy postpartum period as deliberately as you prepared for pregnancy and birth. (Albeit with a light touch and the ability to adapt; as with anything child-related, we know that nothing ever goes quite to plan.) It is a book for the mother-to-be to read before the baby comes and afterward, in the snippets of time she might have between feeding and rocking. Just as important, it is for the people who love the mother and her child and who want to show up for both of them in the most helpful ways they can.

The spectrum of women's experiences is wide after childbirth, encompassing the woman with minimal maternity leave and the one who plans to stay home indefinitely. But pretty much everyone experiences how the first forty days are inherently imperfect, rife with confusing and clumsy moments, dotted with messy and awkward parts, and sometimes even streaked with melancholy. If you can create space for all the ups and downs, including challenging feelings, and if you can do just a few small things to take good care of yourself during this time, you can help to create the conditions recommended by the old wise ones. You can enjoy a safe, supportive, healing environment that benefits mother and baby today and in the future, and practice staying connected to yourself even while taking care of another. The transition into motherhood—or motherhood again—is an incredibly important time of your life, and there is always an opportunity to bring sacredness into the experience of caring for a new baby. Even if you didn't enjoy it with your first child, or your second, this book serves to make sacredness part of your mothering experience now.

Our generation is in the middle of a grand rethinking about how we birth and how we mother. Through sharing our personal experiences about pregnancy, birth, and parenting without reserve—in mothers' groups and online forums—we are moving toward a new way of mothering that is more thoughtful and authentic, and that reconsiders what we and our children truly need. In a society that applies pressure from all sides to be faster and more productive, to "bounce back" and charge forward, women are beginning to invite one another to slow down, take a breath, and make choices that meet those needs in a more generous way. Bringing attention and care to the postpartum period is a key part of the puzzle.

This book was designed to be your ally as you move through the first tender weeks with your baby. It was written under the pulsing beat of one guiding question: *What does a new mother need to feel supported and nurtured?* I invite you to lean on the knowledge and recipes contained in these pages and then pass this book on to the next mother-to-be, telling her which parts of it inspired, helped, or fed you best. In that way, the wisdom gets carried on in a ripple effect, touching more women, widening the circle of support. It's time to start a new tradition—a movement—of postpartum care: one that honors the past and that will carry us, and our children, more kindly and happily into the future.

1

my story

My extended Chinese-American family includes quite a few legendary characters, but few can match my Auntie Ou for sheer personality. She is a phenomenon to herself: a petite dynamo of a woman whose passion for her art of Chinese healing is as strong today as when she first began practicing in the seventies. Auntie Ou can diagnose you with a glance at your tongue and her fingers on your pulse. Her no-frills clinic in Oakland, California, hasn't changed a bit in decades. Its jumble of herb jars, meridian charts, and medical textbooks will never need a makeover, because she is renowned, along with my other aunt and my uncle, also acupuncturists and herbalists, for her ability to help women with every aspect of their reproductive health.

Of equal renown is the fifty-four-day stint of *zuo yuezi* that Auntie Ou did after the birth of her daughter Wendy, back in China. *Zuo yuezi*, sometimes translated as "sitting the month," is a very Chinese tradition: a health and wellness protocol that is devoted to the needs of the new mother and that starts within minutes of baby being delivered. Lesser women than she would follow this protocol for a mere thirty days—approximately one lunar cycle—but Auntie Ou, the descendant of many Chinese healers, took it to the next level. For almost two months, she will proudly tell you, she stayed indoors with her newborn, sheltered from cold and wind; she ate two pork kidneys a day to rebuild her *jing*, the life essence stored in her own kidneys; and she dutifully drank whatever healing soup or tea her mother-in-law served. She also refrained from bathing or washing her hair for a whole month, as tradition dictates. Auntie Ou firmly believes that this dedicated confinement care in her twenties—"confinement" is the most commonly used English translation of *zuo yuezi*—is responsible for the vibrancy, resiliency, and youthful good looks she enjoys today, in her mid-sixties. "I took care of myself postpartum, that's why I'm so strong," she likes to say, as her arthritis-free hands deftly cut up a chicken for the pot and her face displays its notably wrinkle-free glow.

This maternal endurance feat was a secret to me as a child. Although I could often be found hovering at my aunts' and grandmother's sides in the kitchen when my brother and I visited from St. Louis, devouring everything they told us about healing with herbs and food, and fascinated by the skillful way they combined ingredients in the pot, I never heard Auntie Ou speak about the ancient ways of mother care. Until the day came that I gave birth myself.

By this time, I was living quite a different existence, six hours south and a world away from my Chinese-immigrant relatives. After graduating from art school, becoming a graphic designer, and subsequently traveling and working overseas, I'd settled in Los Angeles to start a family. "Traditional" wasn't exactly a word that described me; "free spirit" might be more like it. I've never liked constraints or been good at following rules. And as a first-generation Asian kid from Middle America with a strong case of wanderlust, I have always been the bohemian black sheep, an outsider wherever I go. I've learned to embrace that—traveling at the drop of a hat, exploring back alley street markets, and merging into new cultures and peoples to discover how they live. This freedom from convention has informed my cooking and my whole approach to business and life. My heritage surrounds me like incense smoke—memories and inspirations guide much of what I design and cook—but in everyday life, I wear flip-flops and I like to surf.

So it was a surprise when the ancient ways of China showed up at my door. One day after my newborn daughter Khefri and I returned home from the hospital's birthing center, Auntie Ou arrived to initiate me into *zuo yuezi* with her grown daughter Wendy by her side. Fresh off the bus from Oakland, their arms were filled with groceries they'd picked up in downtown LA's Chinese markets. Wrinkled chicken feet and knobs of fragrant ginger; bottles of rice wine and bags of peanuts; flaky, jade green seaweed and voluptuous papayas—and the pièce de résistance, some scary-looking pig hooves. They cheerfully yelled at me to stay in my room with the baby and marched into my kitchen to set up camp. With a clang of pots and pans, they began the process of making the traditional dishes that would restore me after birth.

I quickly discovered that Auntie Ou's "confinement care" came with a set of commandments: For one week after birth, I was to eat especially slowly, because my digestion was weak, and prioritize soft, traditional foods like black sesame with rice powder and ginger or congee with black sugar. Absolutely no cold food or drinks were to pass my lips, because these would slow down the circulation of blood necessary for optimal healing. After one week, I could graduate to eating the special postpartum soups they were creating from long-simmered bone broth and fish stock—these would help amplify and enrich my breast milk and balance my hormones so that my mood stayed elevated. Meanwhile, I was to stay in bed—or close to it—at all times, keeping my activity levels ultralow, and clothe myself in thick woolen socks, a cozy hat, and extra blankets so that my body stayed very warm. My computer, cell phone, and even my beloved tower of night-table books were hidden away, so that I wasn't tempted to distract myself when I should be sleeping.

According to Chinese medicine, birth is a shift from a yang state, in which the pregnant woman's body is warm with the high volume of circulating blood

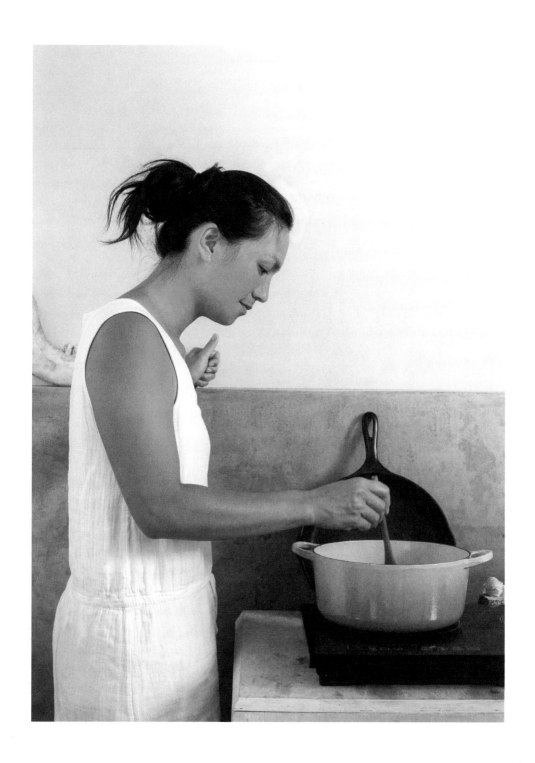

and full due to the presence of baby in her womb, to a more yin state—the empty and cold counterbalance to yang. Women in general tend to be quite yin by nature; after birth, the sages say, this yin tendency is exaggerated, and combined with the depletion in energy levels after the efforts of delivery, it makes the new mother especially susceptible to exhaustion or illness. Exposure to drafty air, eating chilled or heavy food, and overexerting myself would make it easier for "cold and wind"—two of the "six evils" that adversely affect our health—to penetrate my body, said Auntie Ou as she tucked me into bed with baby Khefri. According to Chinese medicine, lingering cold and wind are responsible for many of the maladies that mothers all-too-often report: headaches and period pain, joint pain, and depression. By staying calm and quiet during this vulnerable postpartum period to conserve my precious *chi* or "life force," and by rebuilding my constitutional *jing* energy with nourishment, I could sidestep those disturbances and sail smoothly out of pregnancy and birth and into a lifetime of healthy mothering. As an extra protective step, my feisty auntie clucked her tongue at too many visitors like a watchful guard at the castle doors. She kept a pot of germ-fighting black vinegar on the stove to purify the air as well, just as her grandmother and great-grandmother had done before her for women in my shoes.

Black sheep or not, who was I to argue with Auntie Ou? I was weary, sore, and consumed with getting the tiny newborn in my arms to nurse and sleep. Besides, like most pregnant women I knew, I had invested plenty of planning into having a healthy pregnancy and birth, but self-care after the delivery registered barely a blip in my mind. I had assumed that after a few days of postdelivery R & R, I'd be getting back to the normal responsibilities of life—shopping, cooking, cleaning, working—just with an adorably dozy newborn wrapped on my chest. A modern, independent woman like me, I guessed, was supposed to get back in the saddle quickly. Plus, family and friends would be waiting to meet my daughter. Didn't I owe it to them to be shiny and presentable so they could celebrate with me and claim their photo op with baby?

My aunt's old code of feminine knowledge put the kibosh on those assumptions. "Confinement" reduced my universe to three essential to-dos: recovery, rest, and feeding my baby. As I rode the waves of joy and tiredness and fumbled my way through the first weeks of breastfeeding, I had to unlearn everything I had thought about a woman's responsibility to others. I was humbled by how little energy or attention I had for anything as productive as making a meal for myself—or even making the bed—let alone hosting well-wishers! I surrendered to my aunt's edicts gratefully.

In Chinese culture, food is love and bossy treatment means you care. Homemade chicken soup and goji berry tea are as nurturing as kisses and hugs. The care I received from my female relatives in those first uncertain weeks as a mother carried me forward on a fueling wave of food, and held me in a net of support. When they departed after a couple of weeks—the busy Oakland clinic demanded Auntie Ou's return a little earlier than she would have liked—they left a freezer full of soups, a pantry stocked with teas, and careful instructions to continue this conservative routine of rest, minimal activity, and reliance on my husband and friends to serve me with food, water, and kindness for at least two more weeks, and ideally longer.

Now happy to comply, I noticed how the commitment to slowing down my life had opened a new space for me to hear my body's signals. Chills could be resolved with a pot of warming red date tea; anxious thoughts could be soothed with comforting chicken porridge. The tools I needed to maintain myself were within reach in my kitchen. And, at about week six, I detected a shift: I felt more energized and capable, confident that my daughter and I had found our groove. We were ready to step out from the cocoon and start this mother-baby gig for real—one "baby" step at a time.

The births of my other two children over the subsequent five years brought very different postpartum experiences. My second daughter, India, was born at home soon after I launched a new company. Caught in the rush and convinced I was Supermom—maybe I really had been fortified by the first round of *zuo yuezi*—I literally forgot that earlier education. Wearing India in a sling against my body, I jumped back to my desk five days after delivery, sustaining my business while rocking my infant. Soon enough, though, my euphoria gave way to anxiety and a fatigue I couldn't shake. I had lost connection to my intuition and let my head overrule the signs from my body. Thankfully, the sight of tiny India's sleeping face on my chest gave me a wake-up call. I, too, required a sweet and gentle routine of slumber and food.

After the birth of baby Jude three years later, an unexpected curveball hit my family. My marriage ended and I found myself tending to my little boy and two young daughters as a single mom. Caught in emotional free fall, I fell into an easy trap for the self-reliant modern mother: the belief that as long as my children were safe, fed, and loved, I could soldier through any suffering of my own. Plus, by baby number three, it felt almost embarrassing to ask for assistance. This time, it took the wise eyes of my visiting midwife to detect how this deeply taxing time had invited a "coldness" to settle into my body and my sur-

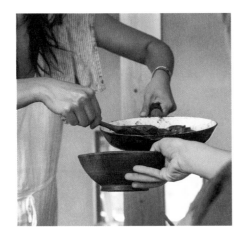

roundings, creating a physical weakness and a sense of withdrawal that she found deeply concerning. Suddenly remembering my aunt's warnings about warmth, and shaken by how little I'd noticed this prelude to depression, I accepted my midwife's prescription of hot soup and homeopathic remedies and rallied the energy to build a circle of support around me. I reached out to girlfriends to request urgent help. These women became my family in this time—a village of sorts—and with their deliveries of food and help around the house, and their gentle companionship, my body, mind, and spirit began to warm up. This time, it took me a little longer than six weeks to find my center again—demonstrating that it can take quite some time for true healing and adjustment to click in.

My three postpartum experiences became my greatest teachers. They woke me up to the range of potential for today's postpartum mother, from being fully nourished in the weeks after delivery to becoming worryingly starved. And they brought into focus a dilemma that goes under-discussed in the excitement around pregnancy and birth. A mom-to-be is surrounded by countless resources and support for almost ten months of pregnancy, but once the umbilical cord is cut, the attention shifts almost completely to baby, and she can easily feel dropped. Ironically, it is precisely this time that her well-being must come first. She is the source from which all life springs. But if her cup runs dry, then nobody drinks.

My mission became to fill that cup for the new mothers in my life. The most supportive thing a woman and her partner can receive in those wild and unpredictable early days postpartum is the thing that can most easily fall through the cracks: food. If sustenance keeps coming, the challenges of suddenly having a baby are daunting, but doable. If it doesn't—everything's tougher. Yet who in this moment has the time and energy to plan shopping and cooking? Too often, mom ends up hunched over the kitchen counter feeling woozy with hunger, piecing together a meal of tortilla chips and cheese, or rifling through takeout menus before exhaustion hits. Though she might have spent months taking utmost care of her nutritional needs while baby was in utero, her well-being often goes out the window once he is out of the womb.

The kitchen became my version of my auntie's healing clinic. I cooked for women I knew personally but also for my girlfriends' friends, giving food to moms however I could. With memories of soups and stews from my first post-partum experience dancing around my mind, I made specially crafted meals with traditional Eastern and Western ingredients to fortify and strengthen a body that is bruised and exhausted, and to encourage lactation and calm the nervous system. My dishes would include hits of inspiration from a trip over-seas, or ingredients that called to me that week at the market. I'd then stir in a giant serving of care and tenderness, ladle it into jars, affix a label, and deliver the gifts with love. (If I could have bottled oxytocin—the hormone of love and connecting—I'd have thrown in a dash of that for mom as well.)

Within a few months, these ideas crystallized into a business: a postpar-tum food-delivery service that I called MotherBees. It proved surprisingly self-pollinating. One woman shared it with the next and our meals soon became popular baby shower gifts—something that would care for baby by caring first and foremost for mom. Sometimes, one or two weeks' worth of MotherBees meals would be ordered by friends or family members as a way of enveloping a woman in a circle of love even when the giver couldn't be there in person. As MotherBees grew, we delivered resources along with the soup, for no extra charge: a sore-nipple remedy picked up along the way, the names of postpar-tum doulas who were available to help, or connections to massage therapists or chiropractors or acupuncturists—or house cleaners!—who were tuned in to maternal needs. We became a hive of mother care that helped women get through their first weeks with baby more easily. Today, the business is expanding beyond California to include a line of healthy postpartum foods in packaged form that can be delivered to a mom no matter where she lives.

When I bring meals to a mother, I try to drop off the food unseen and slip away, leaving her fed but undisturbed. But sometimes I get invited in for a chat and a moment of connection. The women I meet have had vastly different births—at the hospital or at home, with drugs or without, vaginally or surgi-cally. They are living in different neighborhoods, in different marital configura-tions, and with different resources available to them. Many are breastfeeding, a few are bottle-feeding, still others may be receiving breast milk from another mother to augment their own supply. But despite these differences, they are united by a common postpartum experience. The brand-new mom is dealing with change on every level—the shape of her family, body, even her identity has shifted, but nothing is yet defined. She is discovering that despite what she might have thought about the effort of birthing a baby, the period after labor is when the *real* work begins. And it is sweaty, achy, leaky-boobed work at that! It can also be lonely work. In current-day America, partners and family members often work long hours far from home, leaving mom and baby alone for most of the day. And friends don't usually understand or remember what is happening back there in the postpartum bedroom, unless they have very recently been there themselves.

Add to that other common new-mom pressures like taking care of other children, worrying about money, and dreading the return to a job, and the total experience of the first days and weeks at home with baby can feel overwhelming. I have gotten used to exhausted moms opening the door and looking part awed and part shocked at what's just befallen them. Over a cup of tea or bowl of soup at the kitchen table, they might say, half laughing and half crying, "Why didn't anyone tell me it would be like this?"

I don't say anything, but smile and push the pot of tea or bowl of soup closer. Have another sip.

Over the years of delivering my goodie-filled coolers of soups, teas, and smoothies, I've discovered that offering food to the new mom does more than simply fuel her cells. The giving part is just as important. It's an exchange of energy and care that fills her up from the inside, making her feel stronger if she feels unmoored and uncertain; connected to others if she feels alone; and seen for what she truly needs, if she feels invisible or forgotten.

I have also pondered how the scale of possibility for a new mother has tipped so far toward isolation, exhaustion, and junk food, and away from hugs and soothing soups and stews. How did we forget to honor this fleeting period of time after birth and give it special treatment? How did we forget to put a system in place that ensured the community at large, and the mom herself, knew what to expect in the days after birth—and knew that consistent help would be there?

Caretaking traditions that were once second nature have gotten buried, remembered only by the elders in the family, and barely talked about by the young ones. But mothers need them now more than ever before! For one thing, most parents invest endless effort and resources to ensure the best starts for their children. But mothers need a strong start, too. The old ways teach us that the biggest investment is made up front. If mom begins rested and nourished, calm and centered, she can provide the patience and sensitivity—the maternal devotion—that her baby truly deserves. This is much harder to do if she's pushed to the edge of emotion and exhaustion.

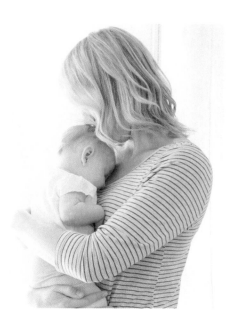

Furthermore, levels of stress, burnout, and depression among mothers—whether they work outside the home as well or are working full-time for the family—are soaring. Customs that insist on rest, recovery, and surrendering responsibility for a few weeks at the get-go force a woman to stop all her doing and simply receive. The takeaway is profound: It can open our eyes to asking for and receiving help so that we can give fully as mothers without giving everything away.

What if we looked at the old ways with creative eyes to see what wisdom they could give us for today? Could modern women approach postpartum with new eyes, not rushing through it in a state of fatigue or stress but enjoying this short season of our lives where we get to play by totally different rules? Could we reclaim this sacred time of recovery and bonding after birth, borrowing from the heritages of our aunties, grandmothers, and mothers-in-law, whoever and wherever they may be? After all, we experience the first forty days only once with each child.

I became fueled by a mission to take back what we forgot and create a new code of knowledge about postpartum care. A mission to support all of the mothers I know now and those I have not yet met; and to pass these ways forward to our daughters, and their daughters, and theirs. Pregnancy and childbirth is the most creative act of the human experience. Bringing a new life to fruition is a phenomenal achievement—some call it miraculous. We need to draw off that creative power to shape a *new* way of mothering the mother, one that works for a new woman in a new time and that gives her the nurturing she needs, but often fails to request. To move boldly forward in this way, however, first we need to look back.

2

from the old ways to our way:

postpartum for
a new world

IT TURNS OUT THAT THERE is an institution of postpartum care that dates back centuries and that stretches across continents. Because this care goes on behind the closed doors of family homes, and is passed on woman to woman—from grandmother to granddaughter and midwife to client—it's not exactly written in scientific literature or discussed in ten-minute doctor visits. You have to dig a little to find it. But it is there. Like a golden rope connecting women from one generation to the next, the protocol of caring for the new mother by unburdening her of responsibilities and ensuring she rests and eats shows up in wildly diverse places, from India to Mexico, from Burma to Arizona, from Russia to Cambodia, from areas of the Middle East to ethnic communities in North American cities. This rope of care is long and it is strong; it holds families—and societies—together. Its individual threads are the millions of aunts, mothers-in-law, grandmothers, and neighbors who have, since time immemorial, shown up with soup and clean sheets and a listening ear to serve the woman who has just given birth.

These global grandmotherly customs have different flavors depending on the locale, featuring diverse but always nutritious foods, from creamy lentil dal to blue cornmeal mush. They have contrasting sensibilities, too. Some treat mom as gently as the newborn, with warm milk drinks and transcendent hot-oil massages; others, like my elders' *zuo yuezi*, have a no-nonsense attitude, seeing this care as an investment for the future—ensuring that the mother's health, beauty, and ancestral lineage endure. But at their core lies universal wisdom about overexertion after childbirth having serious consequences, and constant sleep deprivation taking a toll on mental and physical health. For mother, there was no "returning to normal" right after birth. Far from it.

In its purest form, traditional Chinese *zuo yuezi* advises a tough-love approach of sponge baths instead of showers (to reduce the chance of catching a chill), no books in case reading strains the eyes, and no movies in case sad scenes upset you and disrupt your flow of *chi*—while others take over all your household duties, of course. *Zuo yuezi* is often referred to as "the Gateway," as it is a threshold between one way of being (your life before baby) and an entirely new existence (life with baby). The reward for spending dedicated time in this revitalizing in-between space? The mother can emerge more beautiful and rejuvenated than before. Traditional Chinese medicine (TCM) doctors say that if the woman shirks this recovery, she may experience a yin deficiency, resulting in insomnia, excessive night sweats, hair loss, anxiety, or headaches. Chinese-American families frequently do a bit of *zuo yuezi* without even realizing it. Many a relative has shown up to visit mom and newborn at the hospital with traditional chicken soup, appalled at the idea of her picking at a limp tuna sandwich from the canteen cooler. (A customary gift of dried longan fruit might come with the soup.) That small warming gesture in itself is tradition in action.

In many parts of Latin America, a forty-day period known as *la cuarentena*—it literally means "quarantine" yet also plays off the Spanish word for "forty," *cuarenta*—has female relatives take on all domestic duties to ensure the new mother rests at home, in order to safeguard against future exhaustion-related illnesses or ailments. Her midwife may visit frequently over the first two weeks to check on baby and mother's well-being, and homemade chicken soup simmers on the stove (overly spicy or heavy dishes are nixed). The new mother's abdomen is wrapped in a *faja* or cloth to help keep her belly warm.

In many Native American tribes, ceremony is key: The customary "lying in" period after birth culminates in ritualistic bathing, a baby-naming ceremony, and going to a sweat lodge to boost circulation and help mom's body eliminate any toxins. The Hopi people in the southwestern United States recall practices of twenty-day seclusion periods for mother and babe, during which the mother might be served blue corn piki bread, a ceremonial food. Prepared in an hours-long process by a wise elder woman of the community, the flaky, thin-as-air bread was served to honor rites of passage.

In India, the new mother often returns to her parents' home with her newborn for up to three months of focused care. There, many pairs of hands are on call throughout the day. The women of the family cook soft and nurturing foods, boil fresh milk three times in a row to break down its proteins, and stir in melted ghee (clarified butter) and special spices, so it becomes easy to digest and restores the mother's depleted state. These loving hands also hold the baby whenever mom needs a break. If members of the new mother's family are versed in Ayurveda—the five-thousand-year-old healing art of India—she may drink herbal tonics for energy, immunity, and lactation and receive daily, warm-oil massages from a specially trained technician to soothe her nerves by calming the excess *vata* or "wind" in her system after birth. She even gets taught how to gently massage her little one's body as well—a relaxing and bonding experience for both parties.

Korea's postpartum tradition of *samchilil* decrees a period of at least twenty-one days, and ideally thirty days, of specialized maternal care dedicated to keeping mom warm, snug, and well fed. *Miyeokguk*, a traditional seaweed soup with beef, chicken, or anchovies, is served several times a day, every day, to boost circulation, restore lost nutrients, and enrich breast milk. Gums are tender so icy foods are banned to avoid dental problems later. At one hundred days, the baby is introduced to the wider family for the first time with a *baek-il* ceremony—a kind of fourth-trimester graduation party! This also ends the close-up focus on mom care—she's ready to graduate, too.

Female relatives descend on the new mother's home in the Ivory Coast right after birth. The mother is bathed and massaged in shea butter by her own mother—a pampering rite that saturates skin with healing oils—while her grandmother and grandaunts gently bathe and dress the baby. Younger cousins and aunts cook a delicious meal, and after eating all together, the circle lets the new mother nap, with baby safe in their sights.

In Indonesia, a bright light burns in the new mother's home for forty days after birth to honor the new life that has arrived. The midwife visits daily to massage mom; bathe her in therapeutic baths; feed her *jamu*, a special nourishing concoction of egg yolks, palm sugar, tamarind, and healing herbs; and wrap her belly to support her uterine healing while also checking in on baby. For forty days, the placenta is preserved and kept near the mother before being ceremonially buried. It is believed that the placenta still holds protective spiritual power that can safeguard the new mother from infection or illness.

In Malaysia's *pantang* protocol, the mother secludes herself for forty-four days and receives hot stone massages, full-body exfoliation, herbal baths, and hot compresses to care for the life force that is sourced in her womb. Her mother or mother-in-law may oversee this, or an experienced live-in helper might guide her through this process.

And it doesn't stop there. Ask women of different ethnicities and backgrounds about their maternal customs and the stories keep coming.

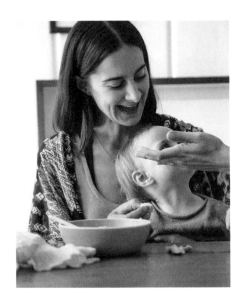

Forty-day rest periods for the new mother are traditional in Jordan, Lebanon, Egypt, and Palestine. The Eastern European country of Moldova has a special chicken soup to encourage breast milk production. In Zambia, the mom is strictly banned from any work around the house until the umbilical cord falls off. (A whopping week to ten days usually—and then it may be back to doing the dishes as normal). Vietnamese parents don't introduce strangers to their babies for six weeks, to protect them from envy or, simply, too much attention. Japanese mothers return to their mothers' houses for a month or two of focused care and traditional food.

In the past, special *pui-yuet* or confinement companions might have been hired by Chinese households to help run the month of care. Modern-day variations of this are emerging, putting traditional programs of postpartum care in reach of women wanting to experience the old ways: In Europe and North America, an emerging field of practitioners known as Ayurdoulas, postpartum doulas trained in Ayurvedic care, can be hired to visit the home over several weeks, bringing food, giving massages, and helping mom learn about baby care. In Canadian cities like Toronto and Vancouver, *zuo yuezi*–trained doulas do a bustling trade visiting homes in Chinese communities, and highly traditional cooking services can bring breast milk–enriching fish and papaya soup to your door. In New York and other US cities, there are even humble Mandarin- or Cantonese-speaking guesthouses where first-generation immigrants who have no relatives nearby can "sit the month" in the old ways with a clutch of other mothers.

At the far *other* end of the scale, in Shanghai and Hong Kong, high-luxury "confinement hotels" offer upwardly mobile women a red-carpet way to experience *zuo yuezi*—call it five-star confinement—and conveniently lets them sidestep the drama of having mother-in-law take up camp in their home for a month. Sumptuously bathrobed in her plush hotel room, the new mom is served medicinal soups from gourmet chefs and can visit an on-site spa as often as she likes, while uniformed nannies handle baby's every need, taking him out for sun baths daily and dipping him in warm pools to tone his muscles. It may be the antithesis

ANCIENT ROOTS

Dig a little into the scholarly texts and sacred books of knowledge, and you discover that this folk wisdom has very deep roots. *Zuo yuezi*'s origins extend four thousand years back in time. The first mention of special care after childbearing was made during the Chou dynasty, and subsequently was written into *The Book of Rites*, which advised the thirty-day confinement after birth—or forty days for twins. Doing a short program of special nutrition, resting, and body care after such a big event as birth was seen as utterly natural; Chinese philosophy says making adjustments in your lifestyle in different "seasons of life" is part of following the Tao or "harmonious way of being"—and doing this well helps you live for over a hundred years! Ayurveda, the ancient "science of life" of India, teaches the principle "forty-two days for forty-two years," which claims that the way a mother is nourished for the first six weeks after birth can determine how successfully she gives her light to the world for her next four decades. And native peoples of the Americas pass their heritage of maternal care on orally, thus making dates elusive—suffice to say, it reaches many generations back.

There is even mention of these traditions in the Old Testament. In Leviticus 12, the laws of life taught by Moses, God decrees that the new mother must "not come into the sanctuary until the days of her purification are fulfilled"—a period of forty days' seclusion and special treatment after a boy, and eighty days after a girl. The exact meaning of this "purification" is a hot topic in theological debate, but the most pro-woman of the readings deem that the "impure" state of the new mother is nothing negative, but simply the opposite to the "holy" state of fertility, and that her seclusion is a protective measure for her and the infant, not a banishment. (The length of seclusion may be doubled for daughters in case they are smaller, frailer, or less prized by the family than boys, thus deserving extra days to boost their health and ensure acceptance.)

The most inspired imagining of this scenario can be found in the bestselling book *The Red Tent*, a fictional retelling of Old Testament stories from the female point of view. In this story, the mother of ancient times is treated like a queen in the safety of the ritualistic gathering site for women—the red tent—where for one month, she is not only nurtured, but also honored for the power of her womb that has brought life into the world. It sounds heavenly—no wonder the Red Tent movement is being reborn in communities worldwide!

A new mother should be treated with massage, warm baths, a specific diet, and herbal drinks that prevent infection, promote vitality and alleviate vata.

—FROM THE *CHARAKA SAMHITĀ*, AN AYURVEDIC TEXT DATING BACK TO CIRCA 400 BCE

During her first month as a new mother inside the shelter of the red tent, Leah was pampered by her sisters, who barely let her feet touch the earth. Jacob came by every day, carrying freshly dressed birds for her meals. Through the hairy wall of the tent they relayed the news of their days with a tenderness that warmed those who overheard them. Adah beamed that whole month and saw her daughter step out of the red tent restored and rested.

—ANITA DIAMANT, *THE RED TENT*

MATERNITY LEAVE
AROUND THE WORLD

The United States is the only developed nation in the world lacking public policies that support women with some kind of paid compensation after giving birth, such as paid maternity leave from their job (and job protection for the duration) or financial assistance if they don't have a job. Other countries offer wide-ranging, and very welcome, maternity benefits—from Sweden's fifty-six weeks' leave at 80 percent of salary to Canada's fifty weeks at 55 percent of salary. In France, a mother gets sixteen weeks' leave at 100 percent of salary, and across the channel in the United Kingdom, she gets thirty-nine weeks off work (with the first six weeks at 100 percent and the remaining at a flat rate). Many nations mandate paid paternity leave, too, and offer parents the choice of sharing weeks of paid parental leave, depending on who wants to return to work first.

of attachment parenting—and it certainly is a status symbol for the parents—but it hits the spot for busy women of means: Every moment of the month is devoted to optimal health for the newborn, and optimal rest and pampering for mom.

This rich tapestry of maternal care through the ages includes protocols that last for twenty-one days, thirty days, forty, and more. What they all share is the understanding that the story of childbearing doesn't finish the moment the baby is delivered and taken into her mother's arms. It continues. If pregnancy is the slow-building Act One of the story, and birth is Act Two—the high point of the dramatic arc—the postpartum period is Act Three, the story's grand finale. Seen through the eyes of the old ways, this several-weeks span is a nonnegotiable time of healing and recovery; it is a woman's birthright, and it is essential for sustaining herself, her family, and society at large. You can almost visualize the woman emerging from her time of nourishment and replenishment—stepping out of the Red Tent or the steam-filled kitchen—looking vital and confident, with a thriving baby on her hip. She is ready to step into her role as the pillar of the family, the one in the center who holds it all together. Informal studies on these protocols affirm this vision: A study on Ayurvedic postpartum care that included short meditation sessions as well showed dramatically higher rates of relaxation, good health, and emotional stability compared to women who had not received special support. And studies of Latina mothers in the United States have shown that even in lower-income families, when the support system of cooking, care, and companionship is in place, infant health outcomes and mothers' well-being improves.

It is a far cry from what most mothers-to-be can expect today. Unless a woman has a close-knit family still living nearby, or is a member of a church or other kind of well-organized group, she probably doesn't anticipate much post-partum support from her community. In the United States in particular, that lack is massively exacerbated by another missing piece: no social safety net of mandated maternity leave or state-subsidized maternity pay. (Yes, scores of nations around the globe offer both—see "Maternity Leave Around the World," opposite.) Most employed American women are forced to stitch together some kind of creative maternity leave out of vacation days, sick days, and whatever unpaid time off their employer condones or their families can afford; self-employed women may have even less backup and require an equally creative (read: exhausting) juggling of balls in the air to keep their incomes and businesses afloat around their newborns' needs. Though it is becoming an increasingly popular area of advocacy, the United States continues to top the list of nations that are disconnected from the basic con-cept of relieving a mother of overwork and giving her dancing hormones the time and space to regulate through rest and proper nutrition. It's a grin-and-bear-it moment (complete with dark circles and wan complexion). And, these days, with more and more women literally and energetically holding the home together as the primary breadwinner, and very often as the emotional center of the home as well, the postpartum period becomes a pressure cooker. The unconscious message beamed from all angles is, "Get back at it. You can't afford to rest."

But it seems we can't afford not to. Anecdotal evidence strongly suggests that when deliberate physical care and support surround a new mother after birth, as well as rituals that acknowledge the magnitude of the event of birth, postpartum anxiety and its more serious expression, postpartum depression, are much less likely to get a foothold. Consider that the key causes of these disturbingly common, yet still highly underreported, syndromes include iso-lation, extreme fatigue, overwork, shame or trauma about birth and one's body, difficulties and worries about breastfeeding, and nutritional depletion, all of which suggests that when we let go of the old ways, we inadvertently helped create a perfect storm of factors for postpartum depression.

It is time to change our ways, to pick up the threads of knowledge that we for-got and weave them into a new kind of fabric to hold the mother. It is time to reclaim the postpartum period and reinstate it to its rightful place as the important conclusion of the childbearing story, something that deserves as much forethought as pregnancy and birth. We must do it for ourselves *and* for our children, because the way women become mothers profoundly affects the way their children awaken to this world. When you take care of the mother, you take care of the child.

the five insights: reclaiming the wisdom

There are five common themes threaded through the colorful tapestry of traditional postpartum care. These are the five insights that remain vital today, by creating better guidelines for tending to the brand-new mother.

1. RETREAT

The ominous-sounding word "confinement" may be unique to *zuo yuezi*—Chinese people don't exactly mince words—but almost every postpartum protocol advises the mom and babe to stay inside for as long as possible after birth and cautions against rushing out into the world too soon. Both parties are seen to be especially susceptible in this time—but not just to the obvious triggers of illness like germs. They're also susceptible to the aggravating effects of cold, wind, and noise, which can penetrate their especially "open" states and burrow in to disturb both physical and mental balance. In Ayurveda, it is said that for a mother to move around outside after birth is like leaving all the doors and windows of your house wide open and allowing the drying and physically and mentally disturbing winds of *vata* to whip through its rooms. Any which way you cut it, the logic goes: lie low. Keep activity minimal and let the mind rest in its simplest form of awareness with few distractions and responsibilities, so that mom's and baby's brain waves stay closely in sync.

Oh, how far we've strayed from that old wisdom! Somehow, a pervasive idea has spread in modern times that the mom who is out and about soonest with her baby is somehow the strongest, like an episode of *Survivor*. For some type-A parents, it's almost a badge of honor to say you made it to yoga after two weeks, snuck off to the office for a meeting, or flew with your infant across time zones. But that's all upside down—in a healthy postpartum period, it's she who stays *still* that wins the prize!

Along with underestimating the need for stillness, modern families also underestimate the need for the space and time it takes to get used to life with

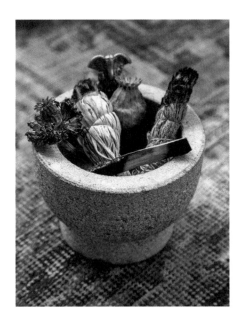

baby. It's not all roses and rainbows with a new-born in the house. Closing the curtains and hunkering down for much more time than you think you need is key to making the transition.

I trade the word "confinement" for "re-treat"—a softer and more liberated version of the idea of staying home. Here, you dial down the distractions and lie low. Retreat doesn't mean lonely sanctum—or as a friend recently called it, "momsolation." On the contrary, it pulses with gentle companionship. When you retreat, you can say no to as much activity and as many people as you want. You get full per-mission to turn it off (be it technology or your tendency to host and take care of others). A mother today might have business obliga-tions she can't completely disregard for forty days, but she can practice restraint—setting boundaries, arranging cover, and forewarning clients or bosses. And retreating is good news for baby, too! This period of rest offers plenty of opportunity to practice shifting the awareness—and gushy feelings—back to the infant in front of you instead of automatically checking your inbox.

2. WARMTH

At the foundation of many mother-care protocols is the practice of preserv-ing and building warmth in the body. A woman's blood volume almost doubles during pregnancy to support her growing baby; after birth, the loss of this excess of warm, circulating blood, combined with her open state, means that heat must be recaptured and circulation boosted to optimize healing. In addition, any nooks and crannies of the body where cold penetrates and lingers—spine and neck, or abdomen, for example—can lead to pain or dysfunction there later in life. To achieve this, new moms worldwide do all kinds of heating and insulating practices, from steaming over hot rocks (Cambodia) to taking herb-filled baths (Thailand) to putting cotton wool in the ears to keep out "bad air" (Honduras) and wearing woolen sweaters even in sweltering summer months (India).

Some of the traditional indictments against cold may not be entirely rel-evant in an era of hot water on demand and hairdryers. But there is one piece of the warming approach that is timeless: eating soft and easily digestible foods in the early days after birth, to support the weakened digestive "fire" and gently help to stoke it. These foods ensure that you absorb as much nutrition as possible and include warming ingredients that boost your circulation naturally. According to Chinese medicine, supporting the digestive system or "middle burner" of the body builds up the blood, which in turn builds good breast milk— it's a domino effect. Overstress that middle burner with inappropriate food, by contrast, and the resulting disruption can lead to excessive sleep deprivation and depression.

Today, postpartum nutrition is still a blind spot. Food advice goes out the window in the excitement around the new arrival. Instead of babying our digestion with simple, warm, nourishing dishes, some hospitals suggest a congratulatory steak (a handy way for them to add big charges to the bill), while others offer cold, lifeless sandwiches and chilled fruit cocktail. Counseling on lactation tends not to include mom's food choices. And once the parents are back at home, it is so overwhelming to even think about cooking that ready-to-eat meals and snack foods sneak in and become staples.

You can tend to your digestive fire and nourish yourself the way your body, and baby, deserve by making extremely simple, warming dishes with ingredients on hand in your kitchen. And just as vital: You can ask others to make these foods for you, too.

3. SUPPORT

What helps put all of this care—warming food, naps and rest, cocooning without errands—within reach? Having some kind of support system to help pull it off. In times past, post-birth circles of support were knitted into the fabric of community life. Family members, friends, and midwives and birth attendants (doulas) might surround a woman from before birth until many weeks after, creating a continuum of care that helped with mom's inner emotional stability and her family's outer stability in the home. No chore would be too humble for helpers—from changing dirty diapers to tending to other children to taking out the trash to wiping away tears (mother's and child's). It was just part of societal code, the way things were done. The new mother was not to be left alone, even if her husband was back to work.

Today, the tides have turned almost completely the other way. The village is elusive for most. Neighbors are often strangers, families can live many time zones apart, and well-meaning friends can be locked in long work hours and commutes, eradicating free time to help. Our quest for independence above all else, and living closed off from one another, has made the colonial American custom of "lying in," in which neighbors would attend to the new mother and ensure she was well taken care of, a long-forgotten memory. Postpartum support is often found on the Internet, as moms search for advice and companionship online at odd hours of the night.

But this isolation is also a symptom of something we *can* rectify: the "I can do it" attitude that blocks us from reaching out for help. With a little advance planning, a mother-to-be can put out a call for support in the weeks to come, and she may be surprised who responds and how. Society may not offer safety nets any more, but we can start to make our own.

4. REST

Many of the old ways prescribe staying in bed and limiting activities beyond baby care in order to rebuild *chi* and conserve *jing* (or whichever words for energy and life essence they may use in their tradition). Many add rest-enhancing herbs and calming treatments, too.

They knew that there is no getting away from the fact that the sheer energetic expenditure of recovery and newborn care accrues for every single woman, even the ones who have straightforward births. And if this expenditure is not met with enough rest and quiet, it leaves a deficit that catches up with her down the line.

Perhaps the biggest misperception we have about health today: We underestimate the need for rest and recovery in our culture. In our do-more world, nothing is ever enough and rest is the first thing to get sacrificed. Yet, ironically, sleep deprivation amplifies every ache, sorrow, and stress!

Getting more rest is easier said than done. But it starts with re-orienting our minds and replacing old beliefs of "never enough" with the understanding that recovering and tending to baby, for now, is *more than enough*. In fact, it is everything.

By creating a support structure of people on hand to help, mom will get a little more opportunity for rest; by letting some things go and shifting her priorities, she can recoup even more. Adding in small moments of self-care and room to breathe is the final touch, so that when she finally puts her head down, she can wind down and feel some peace.

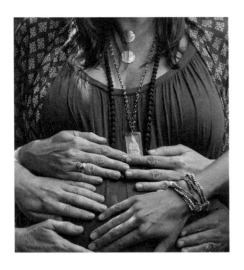

5. RITUAL

Traditionally, postpartum protocols included rituals that marked the metamorphosis that occurs when a woman becomes a mother. They recognized the birth of a child as a rite of passage and honored the effort. In parts of India, North Africa, and the Middle East, women of the community might adorn the mother's legs and feet with intricate henna patterns to not only honor her but to ensure that she would sit still and rest while they dried! On the fortieth day of postpartum in Indonesia, the midwife would have the mother stand over a pot of smoldering herbs to purify her body, and she would give her abdomen a final massage. The infant would be formally named, feasting would occur, and after all these events, the birth would be seen to have been successfully integrated into the woman's experience.

Honoring the mother can be as elaborate as a ceremony or as simple as loving touch. Native American medicine woman Cecilia Garcia, a dear friend, liked to tell me how her people, the Chumash of California, would ensure that mothers were touched throughout pregnancy and postpartum by their women friends and sisters in the community. Their backs were rubbed, their hair was brushed, and their hands were held in a continuum of feminine care.

Ritual and acknowledgment of the mother has always helped to hold the social order in place and let mom know where she is in the larger story of her life. More than a few sociologists have observed that formally acknowledging motherhood as a source of pride and power helps a woman to decrease the fear of birth and stress or even depression afterward.

But today, everyone wants to hold the baby, not the mom! And in the excitement over the little one's arrival, we barely acknowledge the massive transition that has occurred for mother. (The stream of photos and Facebook posts give surface cheer but can't quite capture the depth of what's occurred.) This lack of conversation and reverence can leave a mother afloat in a sea of change, at odds with old friends or even her partner, or sorrowful, wondering if this miracle has gone unseen.

Ritual can be restored to life in small or grand ways, depending on your personality and your energetic availability. It can be as humble as a foot rub given to you by a friend, or as memorable as a mother's ceremony before and/or after your baby comes. It may be the way you choose to tell your birth story to a confidante, or it may be as simple as taking ten minutes to write or draw in a journal or stand in your garden (with baby warmly tucked against you or cared for indoors) connecting to Mother Earth.

The way forward will not involve mothers-in-law or aunties moving in with their cooking pots. Nor will most mothers-to-be reserve a room at a confinement care hotel—neither the guesthouse nor the Four Seasons version. None of these options is in sync with today's lifestyles. The pattern of dutiful daughter (or daughter-in-law) and older matriarchs ruling the roost has changed, and while the elders' wisdom can help us find the way, we are in the driver's seat now. Women today are responsible for a complex web of demands, and surrendering to someone else's law for six weeks simply doesn't fit the reality of our lives. *Our* golden rope of care has to be a flexible one, based on the universal wisdom of the five insights, but offering ease and adaptability in place of elaborate regimens. Importantly, it has to fold in a sixth insight: intuition. It must be oriented to helping *the mother* tap into her own needs, just as she is learning how to tap into her baby's. At the end of the day, nobody knows what is best for the mother and her baby more than the mother herself.

the first forty days: the new way

The book you hold in your hands is a reinvention of some of the time-honored programs for maternal care; less rigid and restricting than the protocols of the past, yet infused with the wisdom that women have shared with one another around cradles and kitchen tables since time immemorial. It is a journey toward and through the first days of becoming a mother. It is free of too many rules and "shoulds" and incorporates plenty of leeway to create your personal experience.

There are so many styles of mothering and so many choices to make for baby's well-being and your own (how to birth, where to birth, how to feed, how to diaper—the list goes on!) that motherhood can sometimes feel divisive. But *The First Forty Days* is inclusive by design. It sees every woman as part of a sisterhood of mothers—no matter what personal choices each one makes along the way—connected by the simple truth that today we must create the postpartum

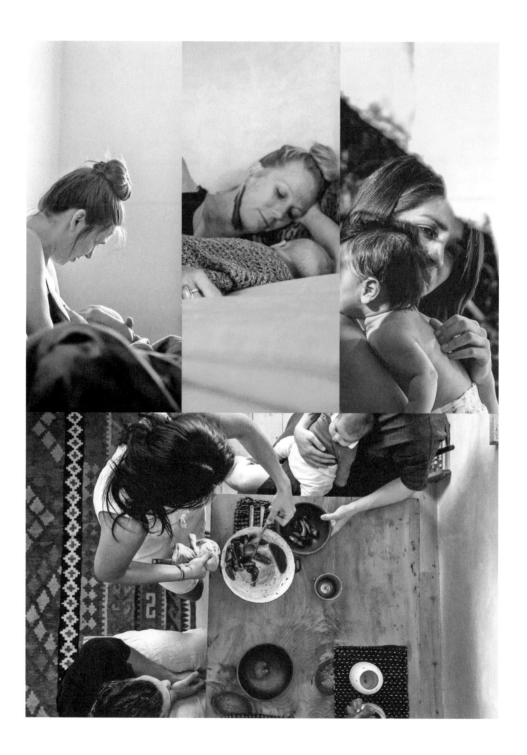

experiences we want. The actions contained in these pages will show you the way. They are small and simple things that you can easily do for yourself or ask others to do for you: make a special warming soup, share a heartfelt conversation, give yourself five minutes for a moment of quiet each day.

The heart of *The First Forty Days* is nourishing the new mother. Eating well can be the first thing to get sacrificed when time, energy, and resources are lacking, yet—paradoxically—the demands of postpartum require you to stay very well fed. You have to refuel after the massive effort of birth while simultaneously doing something extraordinary: creating sustenance for a baby *with your own body*! It's incredible! And it requires energy in the form of food.

Stable and consistent eating is also a preventive measure against emotional distress. Being undernourished and incredibly overtired is a volatile combination. Tensions can rise and moods can spiral downward with surprising speed. A warming meal and a satisfied belly are the first steps to turning that spiral around, or stop it from happening at all.

To do this, I share my postpartum fusion food, a repertoire of dishes and drinks that blend old and new, East and West—the best of all worlds. The recipes take a back-to-basics approach to making simple dishes—either on your own in your kitchen or by asking others to cook for you. You'll discover a range of meals, snacks, and drinks that are quick to make, support your digestion, and fortify you with necessary nutrition. This is a folksy style of cooking that doesn't require much skill or many traditional or specialty ingredients. It is healing food made simply and colored with love.

One important consideration before we begin: Please know that your first forty days are *not* a time to worry about losing so-called baby weight. Dieting to lose excess pounds may or may not be something you engage in during the months to come, but for this tender early period—remember, forty days is not even half of your baby's "fourth trimester"—your onus is to feed yourself wisely and well. In the first phase of life with your child, your body is still shared and your choices affect two people deeply. The good, healthy fats featured in the recipes fuel your metabolism to work efficiently and stabilize your mood. Eating in this way supports lactation, helping your body engage in the energy-intensive act of breastfeeding. So my invitation is to give up fighting with food or stressing about it. I want mothers to enjoy food as nourishment, as medicine, as comfort and, of course, as a gift offered with love from a person who cares.

Around this central hub of food, *The First Forty Days* will invite you to consider the other steps you can take to ensure that you don't lose yourself as you care for your baby—and your partner and other children, if you have them.

how to use this guide

Your postpartum experience actually begins in your third trimester of pregnancy. For the first forty days, the end of pregnancy is actually the beginning of the story.

You will start out in the Gathering phase, which takes place in the third trimester. This is a time of activity and preparation for birth and postpartum. You will assemble your supplies and ready yourself and your home for what is to come.

Then you will inevitably enter the Passage, the short but intense period of labor and delivery that is the bridge between the old you without a child, and the new you as a mother. The information here will assist you in staying fueled, hydrated, and grounded during this extraordinary event.

Finally, you will sink into the Gateway, or the first forty days—the main event covered here and the heart of the book! The recipes collected and the wisdom shared in this section will help you move through this rare season of your life touched by all five of the ancient insights: retreat, warmth, support, rest, and ritual.

Note: In this book, the gender-neutral word "partner" is used to connote the baby's other parent instead of "father" or "dad." Families are composed in so many ways today: the second parent may be another mother, a baby may arrive to two fathers, or there may be no partner at all. The intention with this choice of wording is to make this information as relevant to as many new parents as possible, so that the early days of parenting are as supported as they can possibly be.

As you read through the next four chapters, take what you will and do as much or as little as you like. Choose a recipe that will strengthen and warm you; make a pot of tea to nourish you from within; or take just a word of wisdom to hold onto if you falter or doubt. How you use *The First Forty Days* is up to you.

This book suggests a longer period of maternal care than *zuo yuezi*'s traditional thirty-day program. Forty days loosely correlates with the standard definition of postpartum as the six-week period after labor and delivery when mother's primary healing and recovery take place. Forty days also tends to be a marker when many women begin to want to venture out into the world with baby. And forty is symbolically a very powerful number of transformation. Religious teachings tell us of Jesus's forty-day fast in the desert and the forty-day flood. Significantly and quite wondrously, it is forty weeks from a woman's last period before conceiving a baby to the birth of that baby when carried to term.

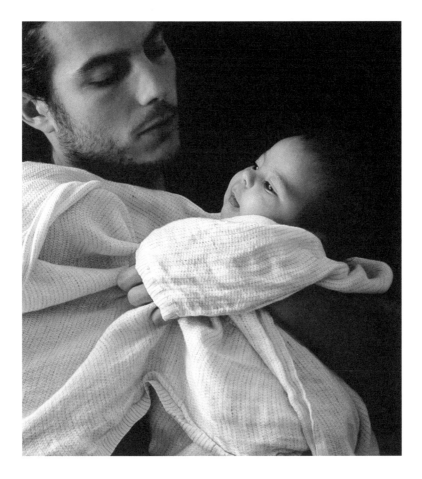

3

the gathering

NEARLY TEN MONTHS HAVE PASSED, and you stand before your future, belly swollen with a life you have yet to know. Baby will be here soon.

As you prepare your home for your little one, a flurry of anticipation moves through you. Your life is about to change forever and you can feel it. But don't lose yourself in the process. Tending to yourself in these final weeks prepartum is essential for your long-term health and vitality—and for baby's well-being, too.

The Gathering phase is an opportunity to build the nest that will carry you through your first forty days of motherhood.

You gather your resources, fill your larder, and create a landing pad that is safe, warm, and welcoming for your baby's arrival, and that will hold you securely as well.

It is also a time to slow down and start to turn your focus inward. Your first tender weeks of mothering will require surrender, release, and tuning into your needs. Start to hone that listening now, and your instincts will be sharp by the time your child arrives.

Birth and parenthood are unpredictable forces. You can wonder and imagine, but you won't know them until they are here. The Gathering helps you turn your attention to the initiation you're about to enter, to ride the waves of unpredictability with ease and grace.

In the final trimester of pregnancy, your baby has shifted from an abstract concept to a huge presence in your life—literally. You navigate the world with your giant belly leading the way, waddling down sidewalks, squeezing into your car or onto public transportation, straining to get out of seats and up stairs. A baby in the third trimester is omnipresent, reminding you that she's there with big—and sometimes painful—movements. You feel each kick, hiccup, and stretch. You watch with wonder as a miniature elbow, heel, or palm pushes you from the inside out. And the world receives your baby, too. Strangers inquire as to your due date, ask you how you feel, wonder if it's a boy or a girl.

At home, your big belly serves as a visual timekeeper, a protruding reminder that things are about to change around here. Especially if this is your first baby, you and your partner are likely feeling the magnetic pull to nest.

You're outfitting your home to accommodate baby, checking gear off a list, prepping a nursery. Naturally, anticipation of baby's arrival runs high in the final months, and these weeks of preparation are an organic extension of the excitement—or apprehension—you're feeling. But this unique time period, this moment before the moment you become a parent—or a parent again—also presents a fleeting opportunity to sink into the significance of your impending tenure as mother. A new person isn't the only thing born on a baby's birthday, a mother is, too (as is a father, grandma, grandpa, brother, sister, and so on).

While you're busy planning for baby, keep in mind that this ripe, fertile period of preparation is designed for you as well. Here, in the Gathering period, you can set the stage for an easeful postpartum experience. It won't be much of a stretch as you're in planning mode already. To make yourself part of the equation, simply expand your inquiry to include the things that *you* may need for a healing, happy first forty days. While there is some very real mystery surrounding birth and those early weeks with baby, thoughtful preparation in the days before will allow you to move into this next chapter of your life feeling safe and supported and more relaxed about walking completely unfamiliar terrain. The Gathering is your time to lay the groundwork for this initial phase of life with your baby. Remember, mothers need a nest as well.

Though you will no longer be made to live by strict rules and regulations like your predecessors, there are some loose guidelines to shaping a successful postpartum period. "Success" here is defined as resting and rejuvenating—with ample time and space to connect with your baby. Food is at the center of it all. During the first forty days, you will eat nourishing foods designed to help you recover from pregnancy and birth, and encourage successful breastfeeding, increasing supply and fortifying the milk itself with healthy fats and vitamins. These nutrient-dense, healing dishes and drinks will be warm, comforting, and tasty, too, and will set you on a path to healthy and energized parenting. The ideal postpartum period will also be anchored by a calm and comfortable environment that will hold you as you rest, recover, and tend to your baby; supportive people who will step in so you can let go of responsibility; a strong and resilient relationship with your partner; and small rituals of self-care that will honor the strength and resilience you've demonstrated so far—pregnancy and birth are significant accomplishments!— while acknowledging your initiation into motherhood and all that lies ahead.

If building your own nest seems like more work, additional to-dos on an already lengthy list, remember that you are baby's lifeline: her source of food, nurturing, and comfort. Creating a safe and sturdy framework for your first forty days is paramount for the long-term vitality and happiness of you both. Do the opposite of what most baby books suggest and put the arrangement of baby's quarters after the setup of your own; even if it's design-magazine worthy, baby won't be clocking much time, if any, in her nursery at first. In the early weeks you will be her entire world, a micro-universe made up of your cradling arms and sustenance-providing breasts. She'll be on you or near you pretty much continuously—to sleep, to eat, and meet your visitors.

As you consider what you'll need to feel secure and prepared during your postpartum period, keep in mind that women are natural gatherers: It's in our DNA to forage for what our families need to thrive. Women fill the larders with supplies for the season ahead, and women weave the fabric of family and community that holds everyone together. Now it's your turn to point this gathering energy toward yourself and fill up your reserves on every level. These remaining days of the third trimester are perfect for collecting the supplies you'll need after you give birth, fortifying yourself with energizing foods, and getting as much rest as you can get. It is also a chance to take stock of your inner reserves and prepare mentally and emotionally for the changes that are to come.

do you deserve the first forty days?

The biggest obstacle to prepping for your first forty days may be your belief system. Though postpartum recovery has a long history, today, simply the thought of making time for yourself or asking for help may seem extravagant, luxurious, or even greedy. *Ask people to cook food for me? Or clean the house? Refuse to accept visitors before I'm ready?* Many modern women are uncomfortable voicing their needs or sitting in the spotlight in this way. But receiving help from others during this time is not a gift or indulgence, it's the natural order of things—remember, this is the essential concluding piece of the childbearing cycle. You're not slipping away to a spa weekend, or seeking out "me" time; this retreat is designed to ultimately serve the whole family. There's an old saying about a mother's well-being: "If there's a kink in the hose, there'll be no water for anyone to drink." The well-being of the entire home—your partner, other children, even pets—depends on your vitality and ability to give.

If you are bumping up against resistance about claiming this time and space for yourself, remember that a gentle, supported postpartum period is your birthright. The five insights are as true today as ever before: All new mothers deserve to enjoy a quiet, safe retreat; healing warmth and nourishing food; help and support; plenty of rest; and moments of ritual. Being denied these basic conditions might jeopardize your long-term energy and well-being, which also will impact your ability to parent the way you desire. Start using this language now with your partner, family, and potential members of your support team and keep using it until you all believe it to be true.

Another way to get motivated is to orient yourself to what the early weeks with baby will really feel like. You can do this by familiarizing yourself with the key factors that influence the postpartum period—and then imagine how you will handle each one and what kind of help you would be comfortable accepting in the process.

seven factors that influence the postpartum period

(AND QUESTIONS TO ASK YOURSELF BEFORE BABY ARRIVES)

1. You will be recovering from pregnancy and birth. Carrying a baby for close to ten months and delivering that baby from your body into the world is a massive undertaking. Your body will need to heal and your mind and heart will need to settle into a new way of being. *Ask yourself: Do I believe that I deserve this time of rest, healing, and bonding with my baby?*

2. Babies require 24/7 tending and, in the early days especially, caring for your little one will be a very real exercise in trial and error as you attempt one way of holding, rocking, and nursing and shortly abandon it for plan B—or C or D. A good amount of your energy will be dedicated to decoding his sounds and movements. Babies can be mysterious creatures with strange—and loud—methods of communication. Sometimes you will succeed in soothing him. Sometimes you won't. Getting to know your baby's unique ways takes time and focus—and patience. *Ask yourself: How comfortable am I with new challenges and situations? Who can I call if/when I get frustrated, scared, or confused?*

3. If you adhere to *The First Forty Days* protocol—and hopefully you will!—the majority of your time will be spent at home during those first weeks. This is a period of great stillness as you recover from pregnancy and birth, and feed and doze with your baby. And after the flutter of initial visitors dies down—a guest list that *you* control (more on that later)—you will spend thousands of hours alone with a newborn, as partners and family members go back to their lives. These weeks are quiet and slow, a curious kind of downtime, yet you will be continuously on call, responding quickly to baby's demands. *Ask yourself: How will it feel to be alone with a tiny baby? How will it feel to step out of the business of my life and do very little? Who can I turn to on good days, and who will be there on days when I'm feeling blue?*

4. Your relationship with your partner will change. It will absolutely change. The dynamic between the two of you must expand to include another person, one who will be literally attached to you for the majority of each day. Where it was once just the two of you, your family unit is now a triad. And an unfairly balanced one at that. The scales are tipped toward baby, here. Biological design requires that it be so. For your child to thrive, your energy and focus must be primarily directed toward his well-being. Affection and attention once reserved for your partner are now channeled toward baby. And while caring for your infant leaves you emotionally fulfilled—or tapped out, likely both—your partner may often feel left out in the cold. If this dynamic remains unaddressed, it can damage your relationship in the long term. *Ask yourself: How can my partner and I talk about our expectations ahead of time? Do we both have a realistic understanding of what our respective roles will be once baby is here? How will we communicate when we reach our limits?*

5. New motherhood—and parenthood in general—is a study in paradox. You will likely experience conflicting emotions . . . at the same time. This can be a drain to your system as you negotiate the simultaneous experience of agitation and adoration, debilitating fatigue and heart-exploding bliss, frustration and magically expansive reserves of calm. *Ask yourself: How do I navigate conflicting emotions? Do I have someone I can count on who will listen to me without judgment or the need to dole out advice?*

6. Whether you're using the breast or the bottle, feeding your baby takes up the bulk of your time and energy during the first forty days. But the quality and frequency of the food you feed yourself is equally important during the Gateway period. Sustenance takes on added urgency after you give birth and as you sink into the process of caring for baby. Nursing mothers require additional calories to support milk production and specific nutrients to make their milk as nourishing as possible. And all new mothers will be in a deep process of healing after pregnancy and birth. The right foods—warm, nutrient dense, easy to digest—can facilitate the recovery process and put you on a path to strong and healthy parenting way beyond the first forty days. *Ask yourself: Who will make food for my family and me during the early weeks with baby? How open am I to new flavors? Am I comfortable requesting specific dishes?*

7. The benefits of the first forty days with baby will only be as great as your ability to tune into your genuine needs and then communicate them to others. As we are pulled along by the bustle of our lives, it can be easy to break the connection to our authentic desires. We are often cut off from that place inside of ourselves that tells us what we need to remain fulfilled, peaceful, and inspired. We make decisions based on what we think we should do, what others tell us to do, and what others have done before us. Now, as your due date approaches, begin to drop the "shoulds," choosing instead to listen to what you believe to be best for you and your baby. The inner voice that communicates these messages will be your reliable guide throughout the first forty days and throughout the next eighteen years of parenting. The more you honor this voice, the louder it will get. Find the courage to ask yourself what you need and then to make decisions that are right for you and your immediate family, regardless of how they are received by others. (This includes being honest about whether you want a parent or in-law staying in your house after baby comes, and if so, when, and for how long. Be brave! It is okay to set limits.) *Ask yourself: Do I have what it takes to ask for what I need? If not, how can I build this courage? Can I begin practicing now?*

preparing for postpartum:
a third trimester checklist

Now that you've contemplated the changes to come, it's time to actively prepare for them. The Gathering is your moment to do some invaluable preparation in four areas of life: your food, your home, your support circle, and your relationship.

Stock Your Pantry

Stocking up with food for postpartum does not mean loading the fridge with loaves of bread and gallons of milk, as if for a winter storm! Instead, to create the food in this book, you will outfit your pantry with some of the oldest and most universal items found in a woman's kitchen, many of which you may already have or feel comfortable using—root vegetables and rice, spices, teas, and oils. You will get some meat and bones (or vegetables) to simmer into broth, which is a foundation of postpartum eating. A modest amount of fresh produce and fresh or frozen protein sources will round out the provisions. There are only a few exotic flourishes in the recipes—most of which are optional. During the first forty days, eating well means eating simply.

Consider that there will be three main ways for getting your meals made. You and your partner will almost certainly make some of these meals yourselves in your own kitchen, especially in the latter weeks of postpartum. (Most of the dishes, snacks, and drinks featured here can be assembled with half a mind, so the other half can be devoted to baby.) I also highly encourage you to outsource some of the recipes to your helping-hand friends, who can drop them off at your door, perhaps with extra portions for your freezer. And, ideally, you will find some time now, during the Gathering, to prep and store some of the meals, or components of them, so that whatever happens next, you will always have something to eat.

Of course, grocery stores will be open after the baby comes and your stove will still function. But new parents are usually astonished at their limited mental bandwidth and lack of time or energy for shopping and cooking. A bit of kitchen setup today will help you sidestep the most common complication for the postpartum mother tomorrow—a growling stomach.

As you will discover, my approach to postpartum cooking is pantry-led. Though you will find simple recipes to get you going, it's not about having your nose in a cookbook or juggling completely new ingredients and techniques every

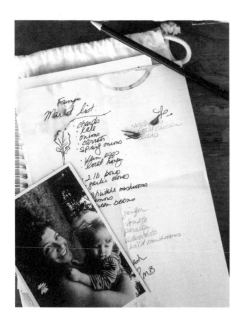

time you want to eat. Who has time or energy for that—even *without* a newborn in their arms? The core *The First Forty Days* meals are built from repeat bases like broth or roasted vegetables or rice. Many of them can be customized depending on what you have on hand or what leftovers are in the fridge. After a few tries, you or your partner or friends will be able to make many of these meals on autopilot. The recipes just get you in the swing.

This advance planning in the kitchen will pay back in many ways later. It will save time for everyone, because when you have ingredients at the ready and some meals prepped, you can give short-and-sweet shopping lists to your helpers, eliminating the need for excessive food shopping. It also saves money, because many of the recipes stretch their ingredients, getting maximum nutrition from a few quality ingredients—a secret of wise women of the ages. And having some home-cooked meals within reach will make buying prepared foods or takeout meals unnecessary, which greatly reduces spending.

To get a handle on supplying your postpartum kitchen, I recommend taking the following actions:

- Read "The Postpartum Pantry" on page 110, and stock your kitchen with key ingredients for the dishes you are most likely to make. Starting a couple of weeks before your due date, practice filling your fridge with necessary fresh items for the first week or ten days at home. Use them up, but with an eye to replenishing them.

- Get familiar with the recipes and make some of them now.

- Batch cook a few of the suggested recipes for freezing like broths, soups, and stews, and make snack recipes to store in the pantry or cupboard.

- Ask a friend to set up an online "meal train" using mealtrain.com or a similar method for receiving meals from your community. Some people will want to cook you meals they already know how to make; others will be inspired to try recipes you show them from this book. Most people do want to make you something you genuinely *want* to eat. It is up to you to ask for what you need—use the recipes in this book as an inspirational guide—and adapt your request to the person who is offering to cook.

Organizing these minor details ahead of time will feel like a major triumph as you journey through your first forty days.

fill your freezer

Cook and freeze some of *The First Forty Days* meals now, and you will have won half the battle of staying well fed. Batch cooking a big pot of broth or soup can be a satisfying and contemplative thing to do on your own. But it can also be an opportunity to gather your team and work together to build your postpartum nest. Throughout time, women have gathered in circles around the kitchen table to "put up" provisions in the larder for the season ahead. Call on that tradition today and enroll one or two of your friends—female or male—to come over with an apron and cook together. Sharing chatter, laughter, and stories as you work triggers the release of happy-making hormones, which is good for you, and good for baby, too.

A few suggestions on recipes from this book to make in advance, in order of priority:

1. The most helpful food to have cooked, bagged, and frozen is the simplest one: broth. Whether it's made of chicken, beef, pork, fish, or vegetables, homemade, nutrient-rich broth is a staple of the first forty days that can be consumed on its own, built up quickly with add-in ingredients, or used to make soups, stews, and congee. Just knowing it's sitting in your freezer will take a load off your mind; after a quick defrost, you've got a super food at the ready. Most people start by mastering chicken broth, but if you can borrow an additional big pot or supplement with a slow cooker, you can get a second broth, for example, beef broth, going simultaneously. By its very nature, broth making produces big batches of liquid, and the bones can actually be boiled more than once. The first time will be more nutrient rich, but the second time around will also provide plenty of sustenance. Jars or baggies of broth will stay fresh in the fridge for a few days and the rest of the batch can be frozen.

2. Heartier stews with more ingredients obviously take longer to make than the simplest dishes, so these are ideal to have frozen in portions. They also serve the needs of your hardworking, hungry partner in the early days after birth, providing him or her with a substantial meal, even if you are eating more lightly.

3. Preparing some snacks with long shelf lives like granola, and organizing your herbs for teas and infusions into glass jars, are perfect activities for the last weeks of pregnancy. Mixing the herbs for the body-soothing Comfrey Sitz Bath (page 221) is also wise. It will connect you to the sisterhood of healing women that has existed since the beginning of time! Another extremely satisfying project: decanting your dried goods (grains, beans, legumes) into labeled containers with a sticker, noting cooking ratios of ingredient to liquid, and cooking times. This means anyone who can read can get a pot of food simmering for you when they visit.

shower power

Babies tend to get showered with presents in the run-up to their arrival. But it's time that mom gets in on the love as well. If you dare, add some utilitarian "you-centered" items to your baby registry or wish list: ingredients and equipment necessary for your postpartum kitchen. These are gifts that will help you and, by extension, baby, in your early days together. And the pragmatic types who pick up on these cues and actually give them to you (instead of indulging their love of pastel-colored onesies) may be the ones you can count on to show up for unglamorous but essential help with cooking, cleaning, and child care.

mom's wish list

- Gift certificate for organic butcher shop to buy grass-fed meat and bones

- Big tub of organic, refined coconut oil and a big bottle of organic, cold-pressed sesame oil for cooking and body care

- Large jar of raw honey and a tub of bee pollen for smoothies

- Super food smoothie powders: raw cacao, maca, spirulina

- A medley of dried mushrooms, including reishi

- Water filter for the kitchen (see "What About Water?," page 55)

- A supply of premade bone broth for the freezer (if mom-to-be isn't going to be cooking it herself)

- Gift certificate to herb retailer for teas and infusions

- Glass food-storage containers (see "Essential Kitchenware," page 123)

- Nut milk bags

- Baby-wearing device of choice (see page 56 for overview)

- Any other essential kitchen equipment she is missing (see page 123)

NOTE: *See Pantry Resources, page 124, for suggestions on where to buy these items.*

building your reserves

Likely, you've been following your own protocol of healthy eating since you discovered you were pregnant. It's never too late to fortify yourself even more, especially to get empowered for birth and recovery. Try out the new foods featured in this book now, while you still have the headspace and energy to notice what you like best and how it makes you feel—information you'll draw on later to make quick choices about what you need to feel warm and sated. In particular:

- If you aren't already including bone broths in your diet, start now. One of the most healing foods on the planet, they will fortify you for childbirth, and their collagen supports healthy skin—great for your stretching belly and your postdelivery recovery.

- Smoothies (served at room temperature) and soups are a terrific way to take in lots of good nutrition in liquid form—ideal for a stomach that is increasingly short on space, thanks to baby's growing body.

- Mother's Bowls (page 167), with their prepped-ahead components that can be served in a flash, prove invaluable in keeping you healthily fed during the busy final days of pregnancy. (They're also great for feeding other children.)

- A Raspberry Leaf Infusion (page 208), sipped throughout the day, is one of the very best things you can do to prepare for labor, as it helps to tone the uterus and supports reproductive function. Drinking a Nettle Infusion (page 208) will deliver energy as well as iron.

- Start to make a gradual shift away from consuming ice-cold drinks and overly chilled foods. Sip room temperature or warm water instead.

create your nest

While a new baby has no regard for the color palette used in his nursery—he won't appreciate the whimsical wall decals or the pricey mobile you purchased spontaneously the day you announced your pregnancy—*you* will have a keen awareness of your space. Within the first few days at home with baby you'll be able to tell if the pillows on your bed are lacking the lumbar support you need for breastfeeding. You will know if your bedroom lamp is dim enough to keep a hungry nighttime baby in a groggy, half-awake state (hint: if you can keep him there, it's usually easier to lull him back into a deep sleep) *and* bright enough to guide you through changing a diaper or placing a tiny mouth on an engorged breast. During the first forty days, your physical environment can dramatically influence your experience.

The Gathering is the time to outfit your nest. You won't have the energy or motivation to make adjustments once baby is here, so establishing a corner of your home where you can hunker down with baby *before* giving birth is invaluable. You will nurse your baby here, sleep here, introduce baby to loved ones here, and even eat here as you sink deep into the restorative process of the first forty days.

The bedroom will initially be the center of your postpartum universe. This room, once reserved for long-lost activities like sleeping and sex, will be transformed into a multifunctional chamber, serving as a safe space for mother and baby—a place to escape the bustle of the rest of the house—as well as a storage space for the ever-expanding accoutrements of life with a newborn: changing table and diapering supplies, baby clothes, breast-pump gear and bottles, and so on. This will allow the rest of your home to be relatively free of baby stuff, which can provide some newborn-free headspace for you and your partner.

Creating your nest is not about serious redecorating, it's about making small shifts to ensure that you will be as comfortable as possible nursing and soothing your baby for hours on end. Use this time during the third trimester to assess your environment. Is your bed comfortable? Does it face a window or piece of art that you enjoy looking at? Do you have the pillows you need to feel held while breastfeeding? Do you have a lamp that can be easily reached from your bed? Either change the wattage of the lightbulb to create a warm, baby-friendly glow (resist the temptation to cover the lamp with a towel or scarf—it's a serious fire hazard) or see if you can borrow a lamp with a dimmer. You may also want a changing table to avoid back-breaking diaper changes and an exercise ball for soothing your baby during particularly restless moments.

Adding a big, cozy chair to your postpartum circuit is a good option when you are craving more of an upright experience. The right chair can be the throne that holds you up in your maternal glory—and sometimes simply sitting up straight can be the antidote to feeling blue. Keep the chair in the bedroom as an alternative to your bed or make it your place with baby in the living room. A side table (even a folding TV tray will do) is key for holding drinks, snacks, and anything else you need to have within reach.

WHAT ABOUT WATER?

You'll consume lots of water during your first forty days, and by proxy, so will baby. Removing chemicals from your drinking water is one of the best "clean sweeps" you can do in your kitchen; this will positively support your body and your breast milk. The options range from simple countertop filters that remove chlorine and fluoride to under-the-sink systems that take out the bad stuff and then put minerals back in. If you've been toying with buying a filter but haven't yet done it, now's the time to act—or put it on your wish list!

CREATE A NEW HABIT:
WEAR YOUR BABY

We've all seen images of mothers from indigenous communities with their infants strapped to their bodies. For these women, keeping baby as close as possible guarantees the child's safety (there's no better way to protect your baby than having him on your body) while also allowing them to use their hands to work—two necessities in cultures where the participation of all community members is paramount for survival.

Today, baby wearing has lower stakes, but the benefits for both mother and baby remain huge. While many modern cultures favor strollers, keeping baby at a distance is a missed opportunity for healing and connection—for both of you. For a newborn, life outside the womb can be bright, cold, and disorienting. But snuggled against your chest and abdomen, baby has a direct line to your center, the part of your body that is warmest. Here, he can also tune into the rhythm of your heartbeat, just like he did when he was inside you, a familiar thump, thump that is deeply relaxing. Tucked in his cocoon, your baby will feel supported and soothed—you may be surprised to discover just how quickly a fussy newborn calms when he retreats into his baby carrier. The benefits of wearing your baby are real for you, too. Keeping your infant's small, warm body close to your heart is deeply connecting and loving, and it also helps to maintain your warmth—a key goal of the first forty days. Most mothers find that having their babies on them also calms their nervous systems, contributing to a more restful and relaxing postpartum period.

Just like breastfeeding, baby wearing often looks easier than it is. As part of your preparations during the third trimester, I strongly recommend choosing a baby carrier and familiarizing yourself with its ways. There are many options to choose from: wraps, slings, ring slings, front-facing carriers, backpack carriers, and more. For the uninitiated, the world of baby wearing can seem intimidating and complex as you navigate popular brand names—Moby, Ergo, Maya Wrap—and a variety of ergonomic possibilities. Newborns are always worn on the chest, but there is no one right way to do this; the only parameters are that you and baby feel safe and comfortable. Different body types will feel better with certain carriers and personal preference will also be a factor. You may have shoulder discomfort while using a sling or be perpetually stumped by the riddle of the one-piece wrap. Visiting a baby store that specializes in carriers is ideal. There you can test the different options and ensure safe positioning with the help of a skilled salesperson. There are also instructional YouTube videos to rely on, plus the guidance of mothers who are masters of the art of baby wearing (ask your friends for demos!). Better to dig into these resources now, before your squirming, sweet-cheeked bundle arrives.

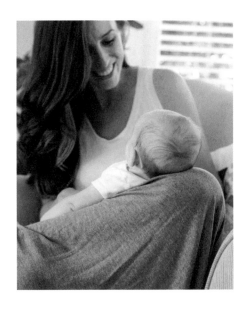

As you build your postpartum haven, check in with your partner to make sure he or she feels comfortable there as well—or is okay with compromising for a few weeks. You may insist on having twelve pillows on the bed or lavender essential oil perfuming the air, but remember that you will also be bonding as a family during these days—and beyond—and his or her happiness matters, too.

Readying your postpartum retreat also includes an overhaul of your beauty regimen. Weed out any highly perfumed cosmetics, bathing, and skin products and set them aside for now. You and baby will be bonding powerfully through smell—of your skin, sweat, breast milk, and saliva, and her skin and bodily fluids, too—and she'll be nestled up against your body, neck, and hair. Let her smell you, not your shampoo and lotion, and shield her from any chemicals that may be in them. In chapter 7, I'll discuss using sesame oil or coconut oil for body care, which sinks into skin to deliver soothing benefits without too much of a scent. This may also be the time to purchase any labor-supporting essential oils that speak to you (see page 76), as well as relaxing lavender oil for the postpartum period. I also highly suggest having the homeopathic remedy arnica on hand to help with swelling and soreness after delivery. One vial of arnica 30c, used per the directions on the packaging, is a good start.

Several unromantic but very helpful additions to your retreat supplies include a hot water bottle for keeping the tummy area warm (if you end up with C-section stitches, check with your doctor first for any special directions regarding direct heat) and the ingredients to make the Comfrey Sitz Bath herb mix (page 221) for soaking the tender skin around the perineum. This bath involves sitting in just a few inches of warm water; a shallow tub (such as an inflatable baby bath) or a sitz bath pan (available from drugstores) are handy tools. A plastic peri bottle is a cheap must-have; it lets you gently cleanse the perineum area with warm water, instead of tissue paper, after going to the bathroom. A cooler left outside your front door can receive food drop-offs when you and baby are asleep or would rather have no intrusion. Or, a friendly note on the door might give instructions for quietly accessing the fridge. Hand soap and a hand towel by the kitchen sink will encourage all visitors to wash their hands well, protecting you and baby from germs. Consider leaving a printout in your kitchen for any helpers who might show up to cook, do laundry, or clean, giving them the 411 on where things are and what products you use.

Lastly, consider the amount of privacy you would like during the early days with baby. You will likely be quite tired and vulnerable, and if you are nursing, your breasts will often be exposed. Would you like all visitors—partner, grandmother, postpartum doula included—to knock before entering your room? Or will you have an open door policy? Perhaps certain times—napping, long nursing sessions—will be off-limits to visitors? A friendly sign goes a long way toward deterring unwanted guests: Quiet, please! New mama napping.

nesting supply kit

- Hot water bottle and peri bottle
- Comfrey Sitz Bath herb mix (page 221) and sitz bath tub or pan
- Arnica 30c, Phytolacca 30c, Belladona 30c
- Essential oils of choice

assemble your helping hands

You've heard the saying, "It takes a village to raise a child." It takes a village to usher a woman into motherhood as well. In the past, a new mother would be surrounded by a circle of caring, doting women—aunts, sisters, mother-in-law, neighbors—from the moment she went into labor and lasting deep into the first weeks with baby. These firm and loving hands would tend to the external pieces of her life so she had the space to melt into the healing, bonding, and adjustment of the postpartum period. But today, we often live far from our families, and that circle of help is not immediate or expected. A woman must be proactive about creating her own version of a postpartum support system.

The good news is that when assembled, this updated village will be the product of your own making. Postpartum traditions like *zuo yuezi*, while undoubtedly comforting in many ways, were probably also a bit claustrophobic for a new mother under the unrelentingly watchful gaze of her mother-in-law. Eeek! Today, you will be able to pull together a list of people that you genuinely like—your mother-in-law may be on that list, or she may not. This customized

If you are employed, the third trimester is also the time to arrange—or confirm—the time that you will be taking off. If you work full-time, you are probably getting intimately familiar with your organization's maternity leave policy—for better or worse! If you have close relationships with clients, alert them soon to your upcoming leave and enlist a trustworthy colleague to attend to them. The goal is to clear your plate as thoroughly as possible so you have nothing to worry about but healing and caring for your baby. If you're self-employed, claiming this time off can be even more challenging because it can feel irresponsible not to be generating income or keeping clients happy. But this is another opportunity to set healthy boundaries, establishing expectations for your absence, creating an "away" email message, even recording a voicemail message that alerts clients to the fact that you will not respond to messages for six weeks (or more). Take care of these essential to-dos now and you'll be able to slip into the haven of the first forty days with peace of mind.

circle, with members handpicked by you and for you, doesn't have to look one way. As you re-create your village, you may find that help will appear in a variety of forms—the circle may be more of an oval. In addition to those who can show up with prepared food or hands that are willing to sweep the floor, do the dishes, or rock a dozy baby while you nap or shower, you may recruit a handful of friends who live in other time zones for regular Skype or FaceTime check-ins. A simple "how are *you*?" can be priceless for a mother who feels herself starting to drown in a sea of baby-focused inquiry.

As you embark on the task of assembling your helping hands, keep in mind that human beings innately want to help. It's in our nature to give back, but you may need to explain the first forty days to the uninitiated, to make it clear that it is a state of deliberate non-doing. Give them this book! It will help them see that in order for a new mother to receive the rejuvenating benefits of the first forty days, she must get as much rest and quiet time to connect with baby as possible. If there was a pause button on her life, she'd press it on day one after delivery and not hit play again until the fortieth day. Have faith that they'll understand and, even if they don't, that they'll see how important it is to you.

One of the most helpful exercises to do during the Gathering phase is to consider what pieces of your life will need to be attended to and who could

WHEN TO GO PRO

Friends and family can be wonderful support people during the first forty days, but they are not the only options for postpartum care. Just as you hire a team to support you through birth—OB, midwife, doula—it's also possible to recruit professionals to help you create more ease and joy in the postnatal period. If you are considering bringing on professional help, use this time during the third trimester to plan accordingly, as most of these positions are booked up to eight months in advance. Whether you're looking for support with breastfeeding, assistance with baby care during the day, another set of hands for nighttime baby tending, or general support for you, the baby, and household maintenance, there are many skilled, compassionate, and experienced people to choose from. They tend to take on slightly different duties in the home, so read on.

POSTPARTUM DOULA: The pinnacle of mother-focused postpartum care. Her primary role is to ensure that the new mother has what she needs to focus on caring for her infant, including making sure she's well fed, hydrated, and comfortable. The postpartum doula also teaches partners and siblings how to support the new mother and gives baby-care tips. They don't have specific duties, but rather step in where needed—doing light housekeeping, checking in with the mother, offering breast-feeding advice, and caring for the baby. Postpartum doulas can work part-time shifts or full days, spanning just a few days or stretching across the first months of the baby's life. Though they may be a bit of an extra investment, this expense may be well worth it to you, particularly if your relatives tend to overstep boundaries and ignore your requests for privacy and personal space. A doula will have no problems respectfully serving your true needs. Specialty Ayurdoulas do this work with an Ayurvedic approach, and include warming Ayurvedic food and massage treatments as part of their care. This may appeal as a lovely, holistic approach to your well-being—treating body, mind, and spirit.

LACTATION CONSULTANT: Breastfeeding is a vast and complex subject. For some women, it comes naturally with little effort. Others will find nursing a baby to be an extremely awkward and painful process. And breastfeeding can differ dramatically from baby to baby. Some infants and mothers are a seamless team, with baby latching on easily from birth onward. Other babies struggle to find their latch and their nursing rhythm. From the start, it's wise to have access to a reliable source of breastfeeding guidance such as one of the many wonderful books on all aspects of the mechanics of breastfeeding. In this book, however, the focus is on ensuring that you are properly supported in all ways as you move into life as a nursing mother. (If you bottle-feed your baby, please do not feel neglected—almost every piece of advice in this book except the following applies completely to you!) A skilled lactation consultant can transform the way you feed your baby. If you are giving birth in a hospital, find out if one will be provided or if you will be receiving one-on-one breastfeeding support from a skilled nurse. You can also line up a lactation consultant to come to your home for two or three sessions. There is something particularly comforting about receiving breastfeeding support in the place where you are doing the bulk of your breastfeeding. The consultant can tell you if your body is properly supported in your bed or chair, and it's often easier to take off your shirt in the privacy of your own home. Thankfully, lactation consultants are often covered by health insurance. Doing your homework now will guarantee that you won't be left alone once baby arrives.

BABY NURSE: A nonmedical professional focused exclusively on baby care. She can work during the day and at night, assisting with every aspect of tending to an infant. Baby nurses can help first-time parents meet the demands of a new baby, while also educating them about the best (read: most effective) methods for burping, soothing, diapering, and so on. Hiring a baby nurse can help relieve some of the pressure that new mothers feel, giving them more time to rest and heal from birth. Women recovering from C-section surgery may find a baby nurse especially helpful, as it can be quite difficult to move around during the healing process, and mothers of multiple births may also greatly appreciate reliable, professional help during the early weeks.

Depending on your budget, you may want to consider additional professional help: babysitters for your older children, a dog walker, a house cleaner, or even a personal chef!

Your OB or midwife may be able to recommend postpartum professionals in your area, or you can search online, as many doulas and lactation consultants have websites. A call to a local birth center or even a local prenatal yoga teacher will almost certainly deliver personal recommendations that you can trust.

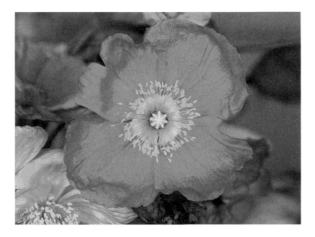

Asking for help can be hard at first, but reaching out when you are in need is a muscle that gets stronger with use. Start now, in the third trimester, and you'll be a well-oiled help-asking machine by the time baby gets here. When you ask for help you are saying that you can't do it alone. But you're not supposed to do it alone—and people want to help. So reach out to people you think would be open to pitching in. A short call or email with a friendly greeting and a clear request is highly effective. There is no need to bury your desire; simply outline it directly and kindly. Not everybody will be able to leap into action for you, and that's okay. But you'll almost certainly be surprised by the receptive tone of the responses you receive.

possibly help with them. Forming your crew of helping hands now, not waiting until later, means the infamous "baby brain" won't cloud your ability to think rationally. (In the early days with a newborn, it's strangely easy to forget who your friends are and feel unnecessarily isolated.) Early preparation also gives your helpers time to gear up—getting some days off work or organizing family schedules and travel.

Though every woman is different, most moms agree there are a few key areas where help will definitely be needed:

Cooking: A mother must have a steady supply of nourishing, replenishing dishes made with fresh ingredients, and her partner and other children have to eat as well. Meals can be made by a support person in the new mother's kitchen or be prepared offsite and delivered. If food is made in the mother's house, the chef must leave the kitchen spotless. Helpers can also commit to keeping the family's fridge stocked with fresh foods. Though texting excessively will prove distracting during the first forty days, consider asking any invited visitors to text you or your partner when heading over, to see if there's anything you need.

Cleaning: A clean, organized home with minimal chaos is a godsend during this time. Support people can help keep the home tidy—or, at least, functional. Those who help will come with a smile and no expectation of being hosted or doted on in any way.

Childcare: It is mighty hard for a new mother to focus on herself and her newborn if she is at all concerned about the welfare of her other child(ren). Trusted helpers whom the children already know well can pick up or drop off kids at school, assist with homework or the bedtime routine, or simply entertain an older child from time to time.

Companionship: Caring for an infant can be lonely work. A new mother doesn't stop being a thinking, feeling person after she gives birth, yet day in and day out with a baby leaves little opportunity for conversation and connection. She needs people who will check on her regularly—to see if she's up for a visit or a chat. They will do so with no expectation, not taking it personally if she says no, and following through on their commitment to show up when she says yes. These supportive folks understand the unwritten rules of visiting a new mother and her baby and follow them closely (see "The Fantasy Visitor," page 165). The need for postpartum companionship extends to your partner as well. Be sure to recruit a couple of volunteers to check on his or her well-being, too—maybe take him out to a movie or for a bite to eat, or better yet, for some physical exertion outdoors, to counterbalance all that time in the domestic cocoon.

Baby care: If you are not hiring a postpartum doula (see "When to Go Pro," page 60), ask yourself which one of your helpers will be comfortable spending time with a newborn. You will undoubtedly need a break from your bundle of joy—time to nap, take a bath, lie flat on your back wearing an eye mask. A trusted support person will take a restless, tired baby off your hands for some time so you can do these things. She will change poopy diapers, bounce the little one for forty-five minutes straight—anything it takes to give you the much-needed rest you deserve. Your infant support crew is particularly important, not only because they will be spending time with your precious child, but also because they understand that the help they're offering is not conditional. It is not reliant on baby being charming and content. In fact, they want *you* to be the one who's with baby when she's in a great mood. They want you pumped up with oxytocin, blissed out, and joyful with a cooing, snoozing, or happily breastfeeding baby in your arms. They will take baby when she's particularly cranky or overtired—they embrace the hard parts so you can catch your breath and take a break.

fortify your relationship

Having a baby may be one of the greatest joys in a woman's life, but it is also one of the biggest stressors on a relationship. Numerous studies have found that marital satisfaction dramatically drops after the birth of the first child. In fact, two-thirds of couples experience a significant negative shift in their relationship within three years of having a child. Terms like "stress" and "profound conflict" are commonly used to describe the experience of a couple transitioning to life with a baby. If you were envisioning you, your partner, and a little one cuddling nonstop in a sparkle of nuclear family fairy dust, the reality of the situation may hit you quite hard. Sure, you're expecting the occasional middle-of-the-night argument and days spent in a zombie-like daze of exhaustion, but genuine strife and possible divorce?

Thankfully, such tragic outcomes can be avoided. With a bit of foresight and preparation before the baby time bomb arrives, you and your partner may be able to keep things in perspective, surviving—at least—until your child's kindergarten graduation. Before you had a baby, your relationship required love and attention or it began to wither. The same applies to life with a baby, but the parameters are different. Taking the time to engage in honest conversation about what your new family dynamic will be like—significantly before your due date—can make a major difference once you're both deeply engaged in the intensity of caring for a newborn. Start by exploring your respective parental roles from a biological perspective. This requires understanding what a woman is programmed to do once she gives birth: nurture and nourish, lull and soothe, with an almost myopic focus inward. On the opposite end of the spectrum, the father or supporting partner is programmed to protect and provide by venturing into the world at large. When living with a new baby, these roles often clash.

Acknowledging your biological roles is first. The next step is to take a close look—again, *before* the baby is born—at each of your expectations about what life will look like when the little one is here. You may find that you are expecting to hire someone to help with cleaning or baby care, but your partner does not feel comfortable with the added expense. Conversely, your partner may be expecting to maintain his martial arts practice—which takes him out of the house two nights a week—or to keep up his extensive business travel while you were hoping that he would be home to help with the baby as much as possible. Bringing these expectations to the table before you give birth will help you find solutions in a

In the third trimester—that's right now!—make some time to ask each other four essential questions that can help avoid unnecessary stress. You may not have the exact answers, but simply bringing these topics to the table before baby gets here can set the foundation for a strong relationship later.

1. How will we divvy up baby-caring responsibilities?

2. How will our finances be influenced by baby's arrival? (This includes the time, if any, that the mother will be taking off from work and any professionals that will be hired to help.)

3. How will our sex life be affected by the addition of a newborn?

4. How will our social lives change once baby is here?

reasonable manner (i.e., when you're not sleep deprived and hormonally out of balance).

For your partner, the first forty days can be a lonely time. A father or partner often feels like he doesn't have a clear role from the moment the mother goes into labor. Allowing your partner to contribute to baby care in his (or her) way will go a long way to making him feel integrated into the family. He may not do it your way, but giving him the space to change diapers and rock a fussy baby in his own style will do wonders for your relationship. It's also helpful to set twenty minutes aside two or three nights a week—yes, even in the early days—to actively connect with your partner. This can look like a calm conversation over a bowl of soup or some focused cuddle time while baby is sleeping. This one-on-one time will be the glue that holds you together during any rocky moments.

And though a woman may seem nothing like her pre-baby self—high on hormones, fluctuating between joy and sadness, consumed with her milk supply, obsessed with rocking baby to sleep—partners must remember that she *will* come back. The first forty days are a fleeting period, and though it may not seem like it when she's sobbing over the empty diaper-ointment tube in the middle of the night, you will both make it through this phase. Just as a new mother can open her heart and mind to include her partner in the baby-raising experience, partners can help things along by supporting a woman as much as possible, without

THE MANY WAYS OF THE BLESSINGWAY

There are many small rituals that friends and family can do to make a mother-to-be feel special and honored. Here are a few ideas for the organizers:

- **Create two lines of women,** one composed of those who are mothers and one of those who are not mothers. The mother-to-be embraces all of the women who are not mothers in farewell and then joins the line of mothers.

- **Invite participants to write messages of love and support** on small swatches of colored fabric and stitch together a prayer flag. The mother-to-be can bring the flag with her into the birthing room and enjoy it during her first forty days and beyond.

- **Ask all of the guests to think empowering or supportive thoughts** for the mother's labor and delivery while holding a beautiful glass bottle of water. The mother can then drink from the enhanced water during the birthing process.

- **Create a foot bath** for the mother-to-be with lovely-smelling essential oils, water, and flower petals.

- **Paint her belly** using nontoxic paints or henna (henna will last longer—if you use it, there's a good chance she'll be taking her painted belly with her into labor).

- **Have each woman bring a wildflower to the ceremony.** Make a crown out of the flowers for the mother.

- **Give all of the guests a candle to light** when the mother goes into labor. They can blow the candles out when the baby is born.

- **Give the mother time to share any fears,** hopes, or concerns that she may have. She can express them verbally or write them down on a piece of paper to be burned after the ceremony.

- **Ask all of the women to sit in a circle.** The first woman wraps a long piece of yarn around her wrist and then passes it to the next woman to do the same. The yarn symbolizes the connection and support of the mother's community. Then pass scissors around so each woman can cut the yarn and tie it in a knot around her wrist while sharing some supportive words with the mother. The bracelets will stay on until the mother goes into labor (a system can be set up where one person is alerted about the labor and then passes the message on to the next and so on). Everyone will then cut off their pieces of yarn and all of the good wishes will be sent toward the laboring mother.

compromising their own well-being. Small gestures like taking charge of an early-morning diaper change so she can sleep in and bringing a glass of water to her when she's nursing—without being asked—go a long way. And mothers can help to keep the tenderness alive in their relationships by acknowledging even the small efforts their partners make. This is often as simple as looking them in the eyes when saying thank you, or a light touch or squeeze of acknowledgment. Or it might be more vocal, with regular reassurance that their partner plays an essential, what-would-we-do-without-you role in this new family unit. And, when in doubt, remember that all misperceptions get heightened and sharpened when you and your partner are sleep deprived, hungry, or overwhelmed.

honor yourself

In the final weeks of pregnancy, it becomes clear that you are on the precipice of an entirely new you. When you become a mother, whether for the first time or the third, you move through a significant rite of passage, an initiation that requires strength, courage, and adaptability. For millennia, women have been recognized for their role in the cycle of life; they have been acknowledged for all that it takes to bring a baby into the world and for all that they must leave behind, and take on, when they become mothers.

Contemporary society, however, is notably lacking in ceremonies or rituals in which significant passages in a life are honored. Sure, we're quick to design a baby shower for an expectant mother, but these gatherings are usually centered around gear for the baby and rarely speak to the significant shift in identity that the mother-to-be is about to experience. Participating in some kind of ceremony or ritual before you give birth is a way to honor the transition that you are about to experience, to bring sacredness and respect to the process of one human being becoming two. Regardless of your belief system or spiritual practice, a Blessingway or pre-birth ceremony will serve as a reminder that you are about to do something beautiful and important.

Traditionally, a Blessingway is a Navajo ritual designed to support a mother-to-be as she prepares to give birth and become a mother. Today, Blessingways can look a million different ways. The only requirement is that you take the time to allow yourself to be acknowledged by others. The guest list can be one person or a hundred, as long as you feel comfortable and loved. You may want to serve teas from the recipe section of this book or the Ceremonial Hot Chocolate (page 216), along with some delectable sweet treats. These gatherings are usually female focused, with girlfriends and female family members coming together around the mother-to-be, but there is no wrong way to do it.

It is not only acceptable, but encouraged, to ask your loved ones for this type of ceremony if it appeals to you. Look at it as another opportunity to practice asking for help!

Any kind of gathering of close friends or family members in your third trimester (whether a Blessingway, baby shower, or cooking party) can be a great opportunity to ask for volunteers to assist with your postpartum to-do list. One guest can be in charge of creating the list of tasks that will need to be accomplished during your first forty days (refer them to the list in "Assemble Your Helping Hands," page 58) and then take names of volunteers for each.

Some ideas:

- Delivering a hot meal once a week or more.

- Purchasing pantry items for *The First Forty Days* recipes or making dishes ahead of time to stock your freezer.

- Several hours of help in the home or doing errands for you and your family.

- Purchasing or giving a postpartum massage, acupuncture, or reflexology (foot massage) session at your home. (Please ensure the practitioner is experienced in attending to the specific needs of postpartum mothers.)

- Making contributions to help pay for a postpartum doula or other professional help.

If a Blessingway is not your thing, you still have instant access to honoring this moment in your life. Simply look down. Finding some time to acknowledge your body—to take in its incredible strength and beauty—is a surefire path to self-appreciation. The curve of your belly, the fullness of your breasts, the thickness of your hair—you are round and ripe, ready for the transition into motherhood. Find a few moments during these remaining days of pregnancy to bring your attention to your body. You can do this while soaping up your belly in the shower, while getting dressed, or while moving through simple tasks during the day. As you prepare for the passage of labor and for the first forty days, appreciate your capable hands, your strong hips and thighs. You may even want to have your partner or a close friend take photos of you now as you dance on the threshold of birth, just a beat away from becoming a mother.

For the majority of mothers-to-be, baby's "due date" is more of a "guess date." Others may already know their child's birthday because they have scheduled C-sections. Yet for every woman, uncertainty and mystery surrounds the events to come. By accomplishing the preparation steps during the Gathering in the final weeks of pregnancy, you have put some structure into the mystery and infused as much order as you can into what is, essentially, unknowable. You have laid down your foundation for postpartum, oriented your mind to the new life chapter ahead, and blessed your body. You are ready—as ready as you'll ever be!—to enter the transformative space of the unknown.

GATHERING CHECKLIST

Have you:

· Stocked your pantry, prepared some supplies, asked someone to organize a "meal train," and passed along a few recipes you'd like to try to friends who are enthusiastic about making them?

· Created your postpartum nest—a space that is both comfortable and accommodating?

· Asked friends and family for the help you would like to receive, and told them how to communicate with you after baby arrives?

· Sat down with your partner (several times) to talk honestly about what you anticipate your new life with baby will look like?

· Seen yourself (daily!) as the powerful, capable, beautiful woman you are?

4

the passage

THIS IS THE MOMENT you've been waiting for—your baby is about to transition from his universe within you to his life in the world outside.

You already possess the strength and stamina you need for this courageous act. It is already within you, imprinted on your DNA, enmeshed into the fabric of your womanhood.

As you transition through the Passage you will not be alone.

Moving into labor will connect you to a powerful current of feminine fortitude, a force that has held women—and their babies—through every step of childbirth since the beginning of time.

Giving birth is one of the most significant initiations in a woman's life, for when a child is born, his mother is born, too.

The bridge between nearly forty weeks of gestation and the first forty days with your new baby is one of the strongest, fiercest, most empowering journeys you will ever make. Whether this is your first baby or your fifth, giving birth is more than a natural part of life, much more than something that just *happens*.

When it's go-time, you will be more ready than you realize. There are many unknown variables in a birth, but there are some things you *can* control. By now, you've likely considered many details of your birth plan. You know if a midwife or obstetrician will guide you through the delivery of your baby. You know if you'll be giving birth in a hospital, birthing center, or at home, and have researched the gear required for a water birth, if that's how you hope to bring your baby into the world. You also have a sense of what your support team will look like. It'll be small and strong, made up of just your partner or a trusted friend, or you'll be at the center of a larger circle of love and encouragement including your partner, doula, and selected family and friends. You may also have a good idea of the support tools, if any, that you'll be using. These can include pain-management techniques, like hypnobirthing and environmental enhancements that can help to make your birth experience warmer and more intimate, like a playlist of empowering or relaxing songs and sacred objects presented to you at your Blessingway.

There are many decisions surrounding baby's birth and there are no bad or wrong ones. As long as the driving energy behind each choice is your own comfort and well-being—with consideration of your partner's desires as well—you can't go wrong. And there are many thoughtful and comprehensive resources that can help you design and prepare for the birth that feels right for you, whether you're leaning toward an unmedicated vaginal birth or you have a C-section scheduled.

This book was created to guide a mother-to-be toward, and then through, the first forty days *after* baby arrives. But to reap the benefits of those first weeks with your baby, you must first take in the magnitude of what you accomplished to give him life. The bustle of third trimester preparation and hyper-focus on the medical aspects of birth can lead to a disconnection from the emotional and psychological—as well as the physical—magnitude of this rite of passage. Entering the birthing process with a reverence for the feminine power that is called forth every time a baby is born will help to fortify you for what lies ahead.

Just as sinking into the healing and restoration of the first forty days is a process of remembering—that this is the way things used to be done, that it is natural for a woman to be held and nurtured in the weeks after she gives birth—turning to a great and mythical source of support during birth requires remembering, too. Within every birthing woman is a great reserve of ancient feminine strength and resilience, an innate understanding that your body is designed to do this, and, when acknowledged, it can serve as a trustworthy guide through the unpredictability of birth. That said, some good old-fashioned preparation helps, too.

THE PASSAGE CHECKLIST

Your birth bag has been packed for weeks, but what about the other things that can help to create an easeful, inspiring birth? Have you:

- Made your labor-aid beverages and packed a few simple snacks?

- Decided on the music that will accompany you throughout labor (perhaps you can assign your partner or a good friend the task of creating a labor playlist?).

- Chosen the inspirational items that will be in the room during the birthing process?

- Purchased the essential oils that will support you? Young Living (youngliving.com) and dōTERRA (doterra.com) are trusted brands.

- Prepared for storing and transporting the placenta?

GINGER LEMONADE SWITCHEL

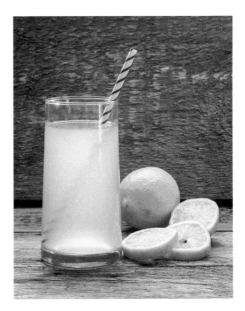

TRADITIONALLY CALLED HAYMAKER'S PUNCH—this drink, or variations of it—was the thirst quencher preferred for centuries by farmers in the fields. Hydrating and energizing, this makes the perfect labor-aid drink. It's also packed with antioxidants, probiotics, minerals, and anti-inflammatory properties. The modern-day addition of trace mineral drops, available at health food stores, boosts the electrolyte value, helping with contractions and energy; Bach Rescue Remedy is a wonderful flower remedy that supports the body and mind in times of stress. This recipe makes about 4 servings. Feel free to double the recipe to keep on hand for natural thirst-quenching energy.

Makes about 1 quart (1 L)

¼ cup (60 ml) raw honey

1 cup (240 ml) hot water

3 cups (720 ml) cold or room temperature water or sparkling mineral water

1 teaspoon apple cider vinegar

½ cup (120 ml) freshly squeezed lemon juice

1 teaspoon fresh ginger pulp/juice (use a garlic press if you have one)

3 drops of ConcenTrace Trace Mineral Drops

3 drops of Bach Rescue Remedy (optional)

¼ teaspoon sea salt

In a small heatproof mug or bowl, add the honey to the hot water and stir to dissolve. Pour into a 1-quart (1-L) jar or pitcher, and add the cold or room-temperature water, vinegar, lemon juice, ginger pulp/juice, trace mineral drops, rescue remedy, if using, and the sea salt.

Keep in the fridge for up to 1 week and give it a shake each time you serve. Feel free to adjust the sweetener and any other flavor elements to your taste.

Often a woman encounters herself in an entirely new way during the process of giving birth. She may encounter the effects of traumas long buried, or she may encounter fear long denied, she may also discover power deep within herself that she had never imagined.

—RETURN TO THE GREAT MOTHER BY ISA GUCCIARDI, PHD, FOUNDING DIRECTOR OF THE FOUNDATION OF THE SACRED STREAM, BERKELEY, CA

Having a baby is a very real feat of physical endurance. You will want to remain fueled, hydrated, and energized to the best of your ability throughout labor and birth. Though there are different schools of thought about eating and drinking during the birthing process—some hospitals still ban the ingestion of any foods during labor and delivery in case surgery becomes necessary—these days, all midwives and most doctors encourage a mother to take in appropriate drinks and light fare if she is craving it.

Electrolyte-enhanced beverages can help replace vital salts lost during the effort of birth and can give a drained mother-to-be a needed boost. But it's a good idea to skip the artificial colors, flavors, and high sugar content of mass-market sports drinks, stocking up on natural, homemade options instead—coconut water is a good choice, but can be pricey. "The Postpartum Pantry" (see page 110) lists everything you need to make your own, affordable "labor aid." Ginger Lemonade Switchel (see page 73), an all-natural, old-world Gatorade that has been used for centuries as a thirst quencher by parched farmers, is made with apple cider vinegar, ginger, and raw honey, resulting in a beverage that hydrates deeply, manages nausea, and soothes the belly with balancing probiotics. Bone broth is another fortifying labor tonic, recommended for centuries as an ideal vehicle for transmitting electrolytes and easy-to-assimilate calories to a birthing mother. Prepping these drinks in advance and having them on hand at your delivery may prove invaluable. Simple snacks (avocado, banana, even smoothies) can also be a boon. But the truth is that solid foods, and even smoothies, do not always stay down; contractions are notorious for causing some laboring mothers to throw up. Sometimes, just a few sips of a revitalizing beverage is all the sustenance you will need to gear up for the next phase of labor.

Though the concept may be squirm-inducing, ingesting the placenta for its super-charged healing properties is another ancient practice experiencing a renaissance. A new wave of naturally-minded modern mothers is giving the organ some very real attention. And you may choose to as well. Retaining the placenta (remember, its delivery is the third and final stage of birth) will allow

IT'S CALLED *MOTHER* NATURE FOR A REASON

Ever wonder why the natural world is classified as a feminine force? Why isn't it Father Earth or Papa Nature? Just like a woman, the character of the earth is built upon a series of notable contrasts: regenerating and destructive; peaceful and cacophonous; ferocious and nurturing. Each of these traits lives inside of us, to be called upon when we need it most. And never will you demonstrate a more extreme range of feeling and sensation than while giving birth. You will tap into your strength and sheer will; you will be humbled and empowered. You will think you can't do it and then you'll do it. And then you'll do it again. Behind you will be the goddesses that fuel the legends, the ones behind the forces of nature, earth, and the universe: Gaia in Greek mythology, Pachamama for the indigenous people of the Andes; Danu in Celtic tradition; Frigga in Norse mythology. As you breathe deeply and allow the transformative power of birth to surge through you, you will tap into the strength of these mythological feminine forces, right into the heart of Mother Nature herself. Connecting with this energy can look a lot of different ways. There's a good chance it will be noisy. Allow yourself the freedom to moan, roar, scream, sing, and cry during labor and birth. Giving sounds the space to move through you can help to mobilize strong sensations up and out of your body.

you to experience its rejuvenating benefits for the initial postpartum weeks (see "Placenta Power," page 79)—and beyond. Midwives around the world, from Italy to Vietnam and beyond, have long encouraged mothers to consume their placentas during a targeted period of postpartum recovery. For centuries, the placenta has also played a starring role in the traditional Chinese medicine approach to a new mother's first weeks with baby. The placenta is believed to support a new mother's recovery from the strain of childbirth, increase her milk supply, even temper mood swings by helping to balance her erratic post-pregnancy hormones. My Auntie Ou tells her childbearing clients that consuming the placenta is the best way to rejuvenate, boosting *chi* and blood.

The placenta can be cooked, blended into smoothies, or dried and encapsulated into easy-to-take dosages. But if you have any interest in consuming your placenta, it's essential to make some plans before your water breaks. You can hire someone to transform the organ into something you'll actually want to ingest (check with a doula in your area to find an expert, or go to

AROMATHERAPY: NATURE'S LABOR SUPPORT

For as long as women have been giving birth, the wise women who have guided them have turned to plant medicine as a natural labor support. Native American midwives were known to use the woodland plants trillium, wild ginger, and blue and black cohosh to encourage a woman's labor, ease pain, and manage postpartum hemorrhaging. Today, some midwives still turn to the natural world to help kick-start a sluggish labor or to reenergize an exhausted mother. Often the plants used are in the form of essential oils, natural aromatic elements found in every part of the plant—flowers, roots, stems, bark, and more—and distilled by steam or cold pressed. These oils concentrate the power of these healing plants into readily accessible form. No need to boil stems and bark into a potent, drinkable brew; instead, you can apply the oils directly to the temples or wrists or apply a few drops to a compress (add three to four drops of essential oil to a bowl of warm or cool water, lay a cloth over the surface of the water, wring out and apply to the face, back of the neck, or lower back). You can also inhale the aroma of a few drops placed into a tissue or add about twenty drops to a spray bottle of water to be spritzed around the birthing room for an uplifting aroma. As you experiment with essential oils, note that not all oils can be applied topically; be sure to read the labels for specific instructions on how to use each oil.

Here are five essential oils that can support you through the birthing process. Some can be combined with others. Be sure to check in with your midwife or OB before using any of these oils during labor.

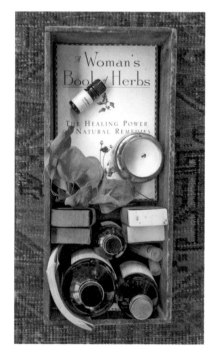

Clary sage: Helps to relieve tension and encourage labor. Clary sage should not be used while pregnant.

Jasmine: Helps to manage uterine pain and strengthens contractions.

Lavender: Can ease uterine pain, increase the strength of contractions, and help to calm the mother.

Myrrh: Helps to speed labor by encouraging the opening of the cervix.

Neroli: Helps to reduce fear, tension, and anxiety.

placentanetwork.com) or you can prep it for consumption yourself. Either way, you're going to have to make arrangements to store and transport it if you're giving birth at a birthing center or hospital. At your final prenatal checkup, ask your OB or midwife about keeping and storing the placenta. They will have information about navigating the specific placenta protocols of your birthing location.

Congratulations, you're on your way! You're as prepared as you can be for the act of birth. But even when you're armed with liters of homemade labor aid, inspirational items for the birthing room, a crack support team, and some practiced pain-management techniques, keep in mind that giving birth still requires a massive amount of trust and surrender. You must believe in your body's ability to bring your baby into the world, tapping into the circle of power created by each woman who has done it before you. And once you have become a mother, or a mother again, you will discover that the first forty days with your baby—and beyond—require the same trust and surrender.

OPENING THE GATES

If the first forty days are all about "closing the gates," the Passage through birth is about opening them. Birth is *all* about opening, actually. The cervix must open or dilate ten centimeters before the baby can move into the birth canal. The vagina must stretch to accommodate the infant's head—and the heart will open to welcome this new child to the world. But if you still feel miles away from such opening, if your due date has come and gone, the ancient ways of Chinese medicine offer a powerful strategy for helping the body initiate labor. Acupuncture can help the "gates" of your body to open so new life can cross through. The acupuncturist will have you rest quietly on the table in semi-sleep as superfine needles (they don't hurt!) stimulate the pressure points that encourage opening. And once labor has started, there are some things you can do to keep things moving along. Ina May Gaskin, a revered American midwife, recommends that a birthing mother deeply consider who she will have in the room with her during labor. She notes that some support people can be "spectators," busy having their own experience while the mother is working to birth her child, while others are "participants," actively supporting the mother with their actions, words, or energies. In her timeless book, *Spiritual Midwifery*, she says: "The birth can be slowed down or even halted until some change takes place in the energy. This is because anyone whose presence is not an actual help is requiring the emotional support that should be going to the mother." This is another opportunity to tune into your intuition, asking what energies will really serve you best during birth.

placenta smoothies

These are prepared using the fresh placenta. Rinse under cold water, divide into six large pieces, pull the membrane off each piece, and cut into smaller pieces, about 2 x 2 inches (5 x 5 cm). Retain some fresh pieces for your first smoothie, wrap the rest individually in plastic wrap, put all the pieces in a zip-tight plastic bags, and lay flat in freezer. When you're ready for another smoothie, thaw one piece under cold water, toss the wrap, then add to blender with the other ingredients. Drink at room temperature.

CHOCOLATE PLACENTA SMOOTHIE

Serves 1

2-inch (5-cm) piece fresh or frozen placenta

2 tablespoons cacao powder or unsweetened dark cocoa powder

2 tablespoons peanut butter or almond butter

1 teaspoon coconut oil

1 tablespoon honey

1–2 cups (240–480 ml) coconut water (as needed for your desired consistency)

Optional toppings: shredded coconut, goji berries, cacao nibs, or chocolate chips

Place all ingredients in a blender, adding a generous splash of cold water to thaw the placenta piece if frozen. Blend everything until smooth. Drink immediately.

BERRY PLACENTA SMOOTHIE

Serves 1

2-inch (5-cm) piece fresh or frozen placenta

1 cup (240 ml) pomegranate juice (more tart) or concord grape juice/guava juice (sweeter) or a mix of the two for a sweet-tart combination, or more as needed

1 cup (about 145 g) fresh or frozen mixed berries (raspberries are wonderful)

2 tablespoons organic yogurt or full-fat coconut milk

1 tablespoon coconut oil

1 tablespoon honey, or more to taste

½ peeled banana (optional)

1 tablespoon chia seeds or powder (optional)

1 teaspoon flaxseed meal (optional)

Place all ingredients in a blender, adding a generous splash of cold water to thaw the placenta piece if frozen. Blend until smooth. If the smoothie is too thick, add more juice or water. Drink immediately.

PLACENTA POWER

The placenta serves a clear purpose during gestation—transporting vital nutrients to the fetus—but its powers don't stop after you give birth. Most mammalian animals are clued into the post-birth benefits of the placenta; all of them, from cats to horses to goats, consume it after giving birth to their babies. Though there is little research behind placentophagy, or the consuming of the placenta, the organ is known to contain prostaglandin, which helps the uterus to contract after birth, and the coveted oxytocin (the "love hormone," which encourages bonding between mother and child and stimulates lactation).

But animals aren't the only mammals capitalizing on all the placenta has to offer. A growing percentage of women are choosing to consume their placenta as part of a postpartum regimen of healing. If you can get past the ick factor, which the (truly) tasty placenta smoothie recipes are designed to help you do, ingesting the placenta can be a key part of your postpartum rejuvenation. In addition to the shots of prostaglandin and oxytocin, the placenta can also help replenish nutrients lost during pregnancy and birth (including iron, which is essential for new mothers), decrease post-birth bleeding, and elevate mood—keeping postpartum depression at bay. The power of the placenta is often quite direct. Many partners note that they can tell when the new mother has skipped her daily dose.

While you were pregnant, the placenta was the nutrient transport system for your growing baby, and it also managed the production and regulation of hormones and opiates. One standout placental hormone is CRH (corticotropin-releasing hormone), which is linked to stress reduction. CRH is usually in the jurisdiction of the hypothalamus, but during pregnancy, the placenta produces large amounts of CRH, which remain in the organ even after birth. Placenta-eating proponents believe that consuming the organ in the days following birth will stabilize a woman's CRH levels, resulting in a less anxious mothering experience.

Interested in experiencing the power of the placenta? You have several consumption options. You can have it cut into 2-inch (5-cm) pieces and frozen to be added to a smoothie each day after birth until it's all consumed, or you can have it encapsulated by someone skilled in the art of transforming your placenta into easy-to-swallow capsules. Encapsulation involves several steps: The placenta is first steamed (many encapsulationists follow the traditional Chinese medicine method, which aims to balance the extremely yin or cold state of the postpartum period into a more yang or warm state by integrating herbs like ginger, lemongrass, and spicy pepper into the steaming process). It is then dehydrated and finally ground and placed into capsules. The placenta capsules can be stored in the refrigerator for weeks. Sections of the placenta can also be made into a potent tincture that will keep for years—some women use it for fortifying themselves before conceiving their next child. As with any supplement, check with your encapsulationist about the correct dosage and notice your body's reaction—in rare cases, women find the capsules to be hyperstimulating.

Consuming the placenta can be a powerful way to close the circle of pregnancy and birth. The organ was created by your pregnant body to sustain your baby, and now your postnatal body, and the baby it still sustains, will thrive from its powerful benefits.

5

the gateway:

the first forty days

YOU HAVE ARRIVED ON THE OTHER SIDE. After forty or so weeks of anticipation, you have delivered your baby in the single biggest act of giving you will ever perform. In one fierce exhale, your child crossed from within to without.

You have both landed in a radically new place. She's navigating a startling universe of lights, sounds, and gazing faces. You're settling into a body that has stretched beyond comprehension, a heart space that is expanding, and a family that has been forever reconfigured. As you take your first faltering, tender steps as mother and child, you are equally raw and vulnerable.

The Gateway allows you forty days to find your footing and inch your way into this new chapter of your life. It is a time and place apart from the outside world and life as you once knew it. It holds you as you recover from pregnancy and birth and as you begin to learn about your new baby. It is a cocoon in which to take pause before the long journey of parenting begins.

It is the great inhale after the great exhale.

In these first forty days after delivery, it can seem as if all the world wants to come and hold your baby.

But to fully inhabit your new role as mother—with its astonishing requirements for giving energy, attention, and love—it is you who must be held.

The Gateway invites you to sink into stillness, and receive.

You and your baby are finally here together. Though the cord that connects you has been cut, the link between you two is rich and vital, pulsing with an intensity beyond any relationship you have had before. Much of the way you move around each other may be instinctual. Baby is driven by innate impulses that drive him to seek your breast and cry out when he is in need. And the way you tend to this new little being may be natural, too. You quickly become attuned to his different sounds, his signs and signals. This most primal introduction, of mother to child, may be the most organic thing in the world.

Or it may not. In these early days, chances are good that you'll experience a stunning range of emotions. Even for the most savvy and prepared new mother, parenting a newborn is fraught with unseen challenges and tests. When a tiny baby is the other party, the getting-to-know-you process is as bumpy and confusing as it is blissful and fulfilling.

How could it not be? Tending to the needs of an infant is a task of monumental proportions! It is one of the hardest jobs you could sign up for, requiring 24/7 vigilance and unwavering dedication. It's rife with occupational hazards, like sleep deprivation, chafed nipples, and teary arguments with your partner about swaddling techniques. The stakes are real, and emotions run high as the most basic questions of survival are addressed: Is baby eating enough? Am I producing adequate milk? Is she peeing and pooping like she's supposed to? Is she napping regularly? Are we bonding correctly? What is "bonding" anyway? And is it normal to feel this exhausted, anxious, or afraid?

In an unfair twist of biology, one person got the job of CEO, COO, head chef, and clean-up crew: Mom. You are the one on the front lines caring for this helpless little creature and the one asking the big questions. But you haven't arrived at this moment rested and rejuvenated. On the contrary. You have just completed one of the most miraculous feats possible for a female human being: You made another person. You carried this baby inside you for over nine months, giving your blood and body to this creation. And then you labored and delivered, a physical and emotional endurance test and powerful rite of passage that is almost certainly beyond any you've experienced.

While you were pregnant, caring for yourself and caring for baby were one and the same. Now that baby has arrived, you must balance your own recovery from pregnancy and birth—and your adjustment to life with a newborn—with the consistent and demanding attention that your baby requires. As your role as mother, or mother again if you have other children, begins, you will quickly discover that the multifaceted nature of this challenge is endless. Though you have just expended a massive amount of energy, you must now source even *more* as you recover physically, orient yourself to a changed body and reconfigured way of being, and navigate the challenges of feeding and soothing a baby.

This unique period of time is called the Gateway because it is the threshold between one world and another. The concept of a pause between chapters may seem strange or foreign, but look deeper—it is as natural and needed as the inhale before the exhale. Forty days of holding the greater world at bay creates a safe space to recover physically, rest deeply, and psychologically integrate the newness that defines those first weeks with baby. Because for the new mother, nothing is as it was before. Time has taken a strange and formless shape, with darkness blending into light as she feeds, changes, and rocks her baby. Her body

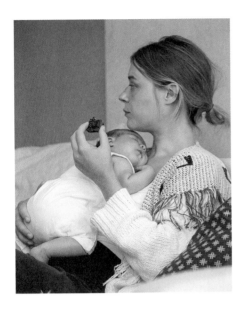

has become an unfamiliar land—unpredictably sweaty, bloated, and sore, with breasts suddenly swelling with milk. Her capacity for even the littlest things, like getting out of bed and taking a shower, might be severely diminished.

And the experiences she had during pregnancy and birth may have left her mentally and emotionally shaken. Chinese lore says that if the complex thoughts and feelings that come up after birth are left unaddressed, or are suppressed under waves of busyness and distraction, *chi* will get blocked and illness will set in. Viewed through another lens, this might be called anxiety or depression. The Gateway offers a crucial moment to feel what's *really* there under the surface and to sink, gradually and gracefully, into the reality of a redefined existence. It is a storm shelter of sorts: a haven where a new mother can recover from what she's been through and begin to make her way toward what awaits ahead.

It is also a tremendous launching pad. According to the principles of *zuo yuezi*, birth is one of three moments in a woman's life, after puberty and before menopause, when she is most open and changing. This openness can certainly cause increased susceptibility to fatigue or illness if not respected. But, it can also allow for a wonderful blossoming as the purification and replenishment after birth reveal greater beauty and vitality. The ancient ones had the right idea: They said a woman could emerge from her first forty days looking more radiant than before!

During the Gathering, you created your nest—a decidedly comfortable physical space built to cradle you during those precious moments of sleep and during the seemingly endless hours of breastfeeding; you assembled your support team, people to help keep your household on track; and you stocked your pantry, freezer, and fridge with the items you need to keep yourself fortified during these important early days. This preparation was designed to be an anchor during the wobbly, unsure weeks of the Gateway. As you fumble through simple tasks, your brain fuzzy with exhaustion and your emotions ebbing and flowing from your newly unsettled hormones, when you forget to do simple, essential things like feed yourself, this earlier organization is there to catch you before you fall.

Just like you and your baby—and your pregnancy and your birth—moving through the Gateway won't look one way or require you to take perfect steps. It is a space that is yours to define; it contains whatever you are experiencing and helps you make small shifts for the better. You can create this with little more than intention, the setting of some clear boundaries, and a commitment to receive care and nurturing, from others and from yourself.

When in doubt refer back to the the Five Insights of the First Forty Days, your guideposts along your healing postpartum journey.

RETREAT: Draw the circumference of your world in closer.

WARMTH: Conserve, protect, and replenish your life force.

SUPPORT: Receive help from your "village" so you can give fully to baby.

REST: Create conditions within and without for good sleep and repair.

RITUAL: Honor the significance and sacredness of this time.

the four phases of the gateway

Never has time been more of an illusion than during the first few weeks with a newborn. You can track how frequently he cries for food, note how often he pees and poops, but your own days and nights have taken on an elastic quality that condenses your world into a series of newborn feedings and stolen moments of sleep. Days of the week become loosely held ideas and mealtimes and bedtimes, fantastically vague notions. But even though baby has no concept of time, there are enough commonalities between the postpartum experiences of all women to give you a sense of what you may encounter during the four phases of the Gateway. This loose sketch will provide general guidelines for the unfolding of your postpartum universe.

phase 1: a soft landing (days 1–7)

Many women will spend the very first days after baby's arrival in the hospital or birthing center where they gave birth, but as homebirth increases in popularity, a growing number of you will spend those days in your own homes. In most cases, you can start to eat and drink normally right away, though after a C-section you

A WISE INVESTMENT: REST

In traditional *zuo yuezi*, it's said that birth leaves a mother in an extremely open state, more susceptible than normal to physical and emotional strain. With her body aching and her senses and nerves raw and exposed, innocuous-seeming things like a brief walk, a cool breeze, or a thoughtless comment can take root and lead to exhaustion, illness, or depression down the line.

The traditional justification for conserving and building *chi,* or energy, through rest and excellent nutrition is equally relevant today. Forty days of care today is thought to lead to forty years of vital womanhood tomorrow. While mother does almost nothing, her lucrative retirement portfolio—good health and energy—is growing! When you consider all that your body is doing during this post-birth phase, it's clear why preserving and replenishing the *chi*, nourishing the blood, and supporting the hormones in this vulnerable moment is so essential.

In one of the most surprising and under-discussed aspects of the postpartum experience, bleeding occurs at a rate that eclipses a heavy period for three to ten days, and then can continue lightly for up to six weeks. A woman's blood volume increases by up to 50 percent in pregnancy, and she grows a significant amount of tissue; this discharge of the excess is an act of repair and rebalancing that's often seen as purifying—a powerful opportunity to shed toxins from the body.

The uterus is also returning to pre-pregnancy size and position. Chinese tradition says that this recently emptied "baby room" is now extra-susceptible to cold and wind. If the body isn't kept warm enough, there can be a slowing down of blood flow to the area, which impedes the uterus's return to its previous size and slows the release of unneeded blood. The consequence may be reproductive problems in the future, from period pain to endometriosis, or even miscarriage, as well as lower-back ache and uncomfortable menopause later in life.

In the first days after delivery, the levels of the hormones estrogen and progesterone drop dramatically, often triggering a tidal surge of emotions around day three of postpartum, as prolactin kicks in. This signals the breasts, which have been making small amounts of the super food colostrum for baby's minuscule stomach, to start producing milk. This is usually somewhere around the third day postpartum, but could be longer if you had a C-section. Rest assured that the high-fat, high-protein colostrum will nourish baby before this happens. When your milk does come in, it will contain the exact immunity-supporting antibodies your baby needs and barring complications, your supply will be intelligently calibrated to your baby's hunger demands.

Skin cells are busily repairing damage that may have occurred through small tears at the perineum or, after a C-section, at the incision point. The liver is detoxifying any drugs taken during the delivery and the lymph system carries them out, a common cause of grogginess in the immediate postpartum days.

The cherry on top of all this activity is that your brain is growing during postpartum, too. Science is now showing how the regions associated with complex emotional judgment and decision making get measurably bigger and stronger through mothering a child, starting in the first six weeks.

This incredible coordination of physical responses will be supported and enhanced by the food and lifestyle suggestions that follow.

Much of the wisdom shared in *The First Forty Days* was born from conversations with the following people, who graciously gave their time and energy to supporting this project:

Elliot Berlin DC, prenatal chiropractor, childbirth educator, and doula

Vasu Dudakia, Ayurvedic practitioner, Veda Holistic Health

Siddhi Ellinghoven, spiritual teacher, doula, and counselor on pregnancy, birth, and parenting

Cecilia Garcia, Chumash medicine woman

Lindsay Germain, postpartum doula

Stacey Greene DC, co-founder, Evolutionary Healing Institute

Isa Gucciardi, PhD, founding director of the Foundation of the Sacred Stream

Jenna Humphreys, LM, CPM, registered midwife, doula, and placenta encapsulationist

Davi Khalsa, CNM, RN, registered midwife

Angela Kim-Lee, MD, psychiatry (focusing on new moms with emotional issues), member of Postpartum Support International

Jillian Lavender, Vedic meditation teacher, London Meditation Centre

Shell Walker Luttrell, LM, CPM, registered midwife, founder of Midwives Rising! and Eats on Feets

Ana Paula Markel, childbirth educator, doula, and founder of Bini Birth

Marty New, founder of ClimbTime Yoga for parents and kids

Ulrike Remlein, childbirth educator, doula, and Red Tent facilitator

Alison Sinatra, yoga instructor and Goddess retreat facilitator

Marijke de Zwager, RM, registered midwife

AND MY RELATIONS:

Dr. Ching Chun Ou, Chinese medicine practitioner, acupuncturist, fertility expert

Dr. Li-Chun Ou, Chinese medicine practitioner, herbalist

And, of course . . . **Dr. Ju Chun Ou,** aka Auntie Ou, Chinese medicine practitioner, acupressurist

may have to follow special instructions to ensure that gas moves through your intestines, and may be advised to consume only broth and tea at first. Women are often surprised at just how physically beat up they feel, even with a short labor. The twenty-four-hour period after birth is like no other. The first sensation a mother feels will likely be relief: that birth is over, that she did it, that baby is here. And though it may take three minutes for that renowned oxytocin rush to kick in, when it does a mother will be filled with wonder and awe, mostly at the sheer physics of it all—this baby was inside you and now he is out!

When you're discharged from the hospital or birthing center—or when your midwife packs up her gear and heads out—the smoke will begin to clear and the new shape of your family will be revealed. These early, early days with baby may be some of the most blissful as your body surges with the oxytocin released during breastfeeding and when holding your little one close. Or they may be some of the most challenging as you fumble to find your footing on wildly unfamiliar terrain. If this is your first baby, especially, you may wonder, perhaps out loud while nursing in the middle of the night or through weepy diaper changes, how so many women, like, *so* many women have done this before you? During his first days, baby looks nothing like the rosy-cheeked cherubs nestled in the arms of those pretty, composed mothers in cinematic delivery rooms. Nope. While your little guy—or gal—is the most beautiful baby ever born (all mothers think this, by the way), he's also a strange creature with eyes that won't focus and inconsistent, piercing cries. He spends most of his time scrunched up in a little ball—he still thinks he's occupying the baby room (your womb)—doing one of four things: sleeping, screaming, eating, pooping. He's not the ideal party guest, no. Hopefully, one or more of your helping hands will be in your home to assist at this critical time. Let them help! Remember, it's okay for you and baby to be cocooned behind your closed bedroom door for as long as you like. If friends are dropping off food, set your cooler outside your door with a note on the door.

During this first week with baby, you may fall madly and deeply in love with your child or it may be more of a slow burn. Remember, there is no right way to forge the connection with your little one. Though she was born from you, she is no longer a physical part of you. For all intents and purposes, she's a stranger, and you may discover that a very real getting-to-know-you process must ensue before the floodgates of love are released. However it looks, it's important for you and your partner to fall for your baby on your own time. Baby's dedicating the majority of his time to sleeping now, anyway—the journey to the outside world was quite epic and exhausting—so there's no rush.

This first week together will also be when your hormones shift in an effort to resume their pre-pregnancy state. Your emotions may go along for the ride. It's normal and expected to experience some blues around day three—give or take a couple days—of baby's life. The first forty days have officially started, so give yourself as much space, and as much comfort, as possible to feel whatever you're feeling. Your bed or super-comfy chair will be your home base now, your cushy landing pad. Follow your caregiver's orders on movement, but chances are strong that the directive will be to take it slow, slow, slow. Be extremely gentle with yourself as you move around your home. Your body is likely very sore. Simply traversing the path from your bed to the bathroom may feel like walking to another state.

Your primary focus in these fresh, early days is to acquaint yourself, or reacquaint yourself if this is not your first child, and your baby with the art of breastfeeding. Though it is a basic, primal part of being a mammal, feeding another human being with your own body isn't always easy or intuitive. If you are struggling or confused about any aspect of the process: getting baby to latch, questionable milk supply, or pain of any kind, don't hesitate to call in an expert! Lactation consultants are a wonderful resource. They can help you master the physical mechanics of it all while deftly and kindly fielding all of your questions and frustrations and, if breastfeeding doesn't work for you, they should be able to support you in making the transition to the right substitute (see page 60 for more on lactation consultants). Make sure to get lots of vitamin C to boost your immune system and help avoid mastitis. If thrush occurs, a few drops of grapefruit seed extract dissolved in water can be applied to the nipples between nursing sessions.

This first week is an exciting one as you and baby, and your partner, too, begin to discover each other while your hormone levels adjust and your body begins healing from the impact of birth. Here, you are just crossing the threshold of the first forty days, officially at the starting line of the rest of your life as a parent. Though it may be tempting at times, there is no turning back. But thankfully, going forward can be a gentle experience. Soft and warming foods will help! They'll give your still-slow digestive system time to get churning again and act as an internal cozy blanket, providing ease and comfort during the unsettling transition that is brand-new motherhood.

Toward the end of the first week—in some cases it may be later—your pediatrician will probably want to see your newborn for a checkup. This will be a big break from your cocoon. Take it slow, bundle up appropriately if it is cold outside, and come straight home after the appointment. Treat yourself with the same protectiveness that you give your baby.

phase 2: the true beginning (days 8–15)

As you move deeper into the Gateway, you will likely start to experience a range of emotions about this new chapter of your life. Physically, your body is in a deep phase of healing and, though you may still be bleeding, you are starting to feel stronger. This is the period of time when a new mother may feel a staggering amount of love for her baby, but is also starting to sink into the reality of her situation, asking the biggest question: How am I going to take care of myself *and* this little person? Whom do I prioritize? You will likely choose baby. High levels of prolactin, the caregiving hormone, help the process along. Even fathers experience a prolactin rush after several days of living with baby. And as you shift into high caretaking gear, you will need your support team in place. You will only be able to dedicate yourself to the needs of your little one if you are being cared for as well—and in some cases this may mean being left alone quite a bit.

During the second week, you are still in active recovery. The initial soreness from childbirth may have faded a bit, and you may be tempted to get up and about more. Don't. Increasing your activity will show itself in physical cues: your bleeding may increase if you push yourself too hard; you may feel extra run-down, or breastfeeding may become strangely challenging. As you sink deeper into the reality of your situation—yes, this little person is here to stay—you may discover a level of fatigue and anxiety that wasn't evident in the buzz of the early, early days. For some women, living with a newborn will be their first real taste of sleep deprivation (see "The Fatigue Factor," page 187). Lack of sleep isn't a joke. It can lead to illness, cognitive impairment, depression, and cravings for unhealthy snacks. All the more reason to stay as closely tethered to your bed or comfy chair as possible, grabbing sleep whenever it is available. Keep your baby tethered, too: Wearing your baby in your baby-wearing accessory as you move gently around the house will provide calming and reassuring intimacy to both of you.

At this point, baby is pooping regularly, signaling that she is successfully nursing and digesting your milk. Hurray, you are on track! And though you are still very much at baby's whim, providing a nipple on demand, the awkward-ness of breastfeeding is likely subsiding. This is good news as she may be going through a growth spurt about now, nursing with more frequency. Note how she's gaining weight—your milk is responsible for all that!—and allow yourself to take a breath and sink into this new world. At this point it is essential to bring awareness to how you're hydrating. Fluids are a key component of breast milk; you can't lactate without them, actually. Aim to take in 64 ounces (2 L) each day—that's eight 8-ounce (240-ml) glasses. Water is number one, but you can also include other options like tasty, nutrient-fortified tonics and herbal teas (see page 206 for recipes and ideas). All beverages should be consumed warm or at room temperature to avoid the dreaded postpartum chill.

As for sustenance, continue with soft, warming foods (all of the postpartum foods in this book can be consumed indefinitely, so don't worry about reaching a limit on any one recipe) and begin to introduce heartier, chewier options as well. As your hunger increases—nursing is a huge energy output, requiring lots of fuel—so will your desire for more significant meals. The Mother's Bowls (page 167) are simple, filling options for an easy meal.

Your hunger may be picking up speed during the second phase of the Gateway, but your world is slowing down significantly. You partner has probably gone back to work, and the initial excitement that greeted baby's arrival has petered out. You and baby are alone more often now, with fewer distractions and interruptions. This new calm may be a welcome respite from the busyness that surrounded baby's first days home or it may be uncomfortably quiet. The revelations will be small, but significant, now: This tiny human can produce more laundry in a day than an adult does in a week; the poop of a breast-

After you give birth to a child, you are in what is probably the deepest transformation process of your whole life! Be gentle with yourself—it takes love and patience to move through this time. Eliminate all stress factors: events, work, household stuff—even family members! And only have people around you who truly support you, who let you be where you are and express what you need, and who know what it's like to become a mother. People who can let you be messy—because all deep change brings a little messiness.

—ULRIKE REMLEIN, CHILDBIRTH EDUCATOR, DOULA, AND RED TENT FACILITATOR, RATISBON, GERMANY

feeding baby leaves indelible marks on sheets, blankets, and onesies; a properly inflated exercise ball is an invaluable infant calmer.

As you move deeper into the Gateway, as the first forty days click by, you will have to remain steadfast and strong as the primary gatekeeper of your sacred space. Visitors will still come calling; the lure of a new baby is strong. Sometimes, a friendly face will bring welcome relief, but other times, it can be a burden. As you pick and choose who to allow into your home and when to grant them access, remember, this time is yours. Friends and family, neighbors and acquaintances, may try to find their way in to your private space, asking if they can drop by for a quick hello and a hug. But you alone hold the keys to your sanctuary. Use discernment to decide if those people will help you, or if they will expect you to host them (see "The Fantasy Visitor," page 165). It's okay for people to wait to meet your baby, even family members. Ask yourself, what are their intentions: Do they want to truly be of service to me, cleaning dishes if I ask, holding a fussy baby while I shower, or are they actually seeking a little hit of baby love for themselves? What energy will they bring into this haven—giving or taking?

phase 3: your new normal (days 16–22)

At this stage, the clouds have parted as the overwhelming newness of life with baby transitions into a (somewhat) easier dance between his needs and your own recovery and adjustment. Baby is now sleeping for longer stretches of time and is more alert and engaged when he is awake—the adorability factor has officially kicked in. At this point in the Gateway, you are moving into the more subtle aspects of engaging with your infant; beginning to crack his code and understand his unique cues. You two are really communicating now, a divine, wordless language that exists only between mother and child. This time is also when a new mother sinks deeper into the very real repetitiveness of caring for baby, one that most baby books neglect to mention. And though you do the same things each day, your little one's sleeping and eating needs are still frustratingly random. It is natural to search for a pattern or rhythm now, but baby is not ready to commit to one. Every time you think she's doing it one way, she begins to do it another way. Ahhh!

And after a few weeks inside, your world may feel exceptionally small, comprising a few square feet between your bedroom, kitchen, and bathroom, or mere steps between your rocking chair and the couch. The hours may tick by slowly as you spend most of your day nursing your baby (most babes hit another

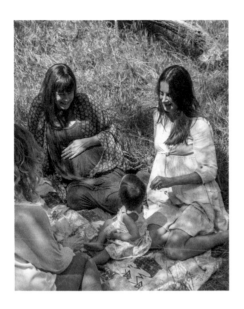

growth spurt between the second and third weeks). Who knew you could spend so much time feeding a baby? You probably feel pretty comfortable with breastfeeding now, but it's never too late to turn to an expert. If any aspect of nursing is still a challenge, don't hesitate to call a lactation consultant.

You may be reveling in the simplicity of your day-to-day life with baby—finding an unbelievable amount of joy in the little things, like the sounds and faces he makes—especially if your everyday life up until this point was fast-paced and overstimulating. Or you may feel isolated and overwhelmed by the monotony. It may seem as if this will be the shape of your life forever, that you will be glued to this chair, your baby glued to your breast, for the rest of eternity. It can be difficult to see past your present moment and to understand that this is a finite period of time, that things will shift and change, that things *always* shift and change. Check out "The Art of Sitting Still," page 133, for tips on navigating all this sameness.

If discomforts arise, gently tune in to their cues. Your body is sending you messages in a direct feedback loop, reminding you to take care of yourself. Breasts becoming hard and tender, even though you've nursed consistently? You definitely need more sleep, and possibly more water (see Tip, page 55). So tired you're wired, even though your baby is finally asleep and it's your turn to nod off? You need something to soothe jangled nerves, such as a warm-milk Sleep Nectar (page 216) along with a hot shower (and how about a back rub afterward with some homemade Rose & Coconut Body Oil, page 220). With small and caring corrections, you can nip many potential problems in the bud.

During Phase 3 you may still find yourself bumping up against a burning desire to establish some sense of routine for your baby, to enforce a sleeping and eating schedule. Try to let it go. At this stage your baby's pattern will continue to shift. He may do things one way for a few days: fall asleep after nursing; wake at 4 A.M. like clockwork; be soothed with a specific lullaby—and then ditch those ways for an entirely new routine. The randomness can be jarring, even infuriating. This is an excellent opportunity to practice relinquishing control.

Letting go of how you think things should be is a major part of parenting, one that will serve you throughout your child's life.

Continue to eat heartier foods now that your digestion is gaining power and your organs are settling back into their normal place. Include a few "power foods" from the recipe section (page 172) in your weekly menu. These nutrient-dense foods feature ingredients that help you rebuild *chi* and blood and balance hormones. And don't be shy about asking for help if it's not coming your way. Reach out to your helping hands with requests for food, company, a foot rub—anything. People appreciate clear requests. Practice making a few this week.

After weeks of stillness, your muscles may be craving a bit of movement. You can do some gentle yoga postures or take a short walk outside, weather permitting. (see "To Move or Not To Move?," page 204). Just be sure to stay connected to your body. Note when it feels like you may be doing too much and pull back a bit. There will be lots of opportunities to move after the first forty days are over.

phase 4: a sense of rhythm (days 23–40)

Congratulations! You made it to the home stretch. You may still be a tad sore, but you have regained much of your strength and are really starting to get the hang of this baby thing. It helps that baby himself is settling into some sense of a recognizable pattern. He is sleeping for longer stretches and is eating during more specific times of the day, instead of *all* day. He may be going through another growth spurt now, showing more signs of hunger, but this will be the last one until he's about three months old. And though other significant shifts will take place, they will happen about every three months instead of every few days.

Speaking of sleep, your partner won't be getting the same sleep-inducing oxytocin rush that you get from nursing in the night. Waking up in the wee hours may have an even more fatiguing effect on the co-parent than on the mother. Be sensitive to the cumulative effect of this disturbance, and do not get hurt if he needs to sleep on the sofa in order to be functional in the morning. This is a good time to check in together with honesty about how you are each faring and how you are working together—and make any necessary adjustments.

During the last phase of the Gateway, you may be mastering the breast pump, so you will have milk stored in the freezer when, or if, you are planning to take time away from baby in the coming months. These final days postpartum, and beyond, will also find you eating a wide range of foods from *The First Forty Days* recipes; remember that warming and nourishing are still the primary requirements.

These forty days are needed for mom, dad, and baby to align their mental, emotional, and spiritual forces and lay their foundation for and with each other. What happens is tremendous: You are building the self-esteem and trust of this new being, giving time for the soul to really "land" on earth and feel safe. If you truly provide that time, the child becomes unshakable!

—SIDDHI ELLINGHOVEN, SPIRITUAL TEACHER, DOULA, AND COUNSELOR ON
PREGNANCY, BIRTH, AND PARENTING, SANTA BARBARA, CA

You and your baby have grown exponentially over the past few weeks—as individuals and a team. You've likely accomplished feats of agility and balance that you never imagined possible. You've probably changed a diaper with one hand—in the dark—with your naked, screaming babe in the other. You've probably nursed your baby while consuming a hearty meal (made by one of your loving support people, of course). And you've probably experienced more exhaustion, more frustration, and more love than any other woman on earth. Except for that mother over there. And that one over there. And that one . . .

As this final phase comes to a close you will find yourself stronger and more revitalized than you've been since baby's arrival, yet still tender and new. This life may continue to feel a bit foreign—you may find yourself longing for the way your body looked before you got pregnant (see "Accepting and Celebrating Your Postpartum Body," page 152) or for the sleep schedule you had before the arrival of your newest family member. But during this time, you have practiced tapping into what you really need in any given moment, setting boundaries with friends and family who want to visit, and asking for help when you need it. You are getting ready to transition to life after the first forty days. Good job making it this far!

If there's a defining characteristic to the early weeks of motherhood, it's that this period is a time of intense paradox. You may experience a stunning array of emotions from true joy—flying high on the oxytocin that surges through your bloodstream whenever you nurse or cuddle your babe—to melancholy, boredom, and despair. Giving yourself space away from social obligations— yes, hosting a roomful of baby-hungry relatives counts—and whenever possible, professional obligations, is priceless in giving these feelings the room they need to move through you.

This gentle retreat—claiming the right to draw your world closer around you for a while and stay home to cocoon with baby instead of venturing out—is the first insight of the first forty days. It is a sacred act of self-care and preservation that allows you to be raw and exposed—literally and metaphorically. Nursing a newborn means sitting semi-naked more than you could have ever imagined you would do—you're letting it all hang out! Knowing that unwanted visitors won't be there to observe you in action will make it infinitely easier.

Claiming your space also means that your new micro-family (you, your partner, your baby, and any other children you may have) keeps the sweetest and most memorable parts of this unfolding time to itself—along with the not-so-sweet parts you might rather keep under wraps.

Most crucially, by saying "Au revoir!" to most of the world, save for your village of support, and pulling up the invisible drawbridge at your door, you recoup much of the energy and attention that would normally be lost to other people and places, and bring it all to the one who needs it most—your child.

For your new baby, you are everything: his provider of food and warmth and protection, his teacher of sleep and settling. You are his anchor in this rollicking sea of stimulation outside the womb and his buffer from it, too. You are his very source of life. Your touch, your heartbeat, your tone of voice, and your smell and taste through the hormones released in your skin, saliva, and breast milk all flavor his first understanding of the world. And he will mirror your state—calm and grounded or overwhelmed and stressed—making it paramount to take care of your own needs with as much dedication as you give to his. You are two people now, but for a few precious weeks that will never come again, you and he are in many ways still one.

6

filling your cup:

what to eat

FOR CLOSE TO FORTY WEEKS, you nourished the baby inside you; now it is you who must be nourished. This is the single thread that runs through the Gateway: putting yourself at the center of the family and making small choices each day to ensure your cup of giving does not run empty.

Nourishment is more than a bowl of soup: It is the sensation of being cherished and sustained. It comes from the way you feel inside your home, or the way an intimate friend sees and hears you fully. But it *starts* with a bowl of soup, because that is the simplest and most satisfying way for your cup to be filled.

My great "aha!" moment about the power of postpartum eating came when standing at a stove in the home of a girlfriend who'd asked me to help cook for a mutual friend who had recently given birth. This was a little after the birth of my third child and—after a rocky start—I had replenished myself and was ready to serve others. I had come without a recipe in mind, but brought a few of my favorite kitchen supplies in my tote, and the new mom arrived soon after. Her several-weeks-old baby was snuggled contentedly against her chest, but she looked anxious and wan. She seemed to be floating above her own body—energetically waifish, even though her body was curvy and breasts were round.

As she sank into a chair we'd pulled in from the living room, cautiously but gratefully handing the child to us for a moment, she confided how undone she felt by the unexpected tensions that had arisen since the birth. Her in-laws had arrived with strong ideas of what parenting and housekeeping should look like, and to her surprise, her husband had not been able to shield her from their damning critiques. It was taking a toll, sapping her of her confidence and joy.

Slicing carrots, filling a pot, rocking the baby, my friend and I listened to her sorrows. Following my instincts, I put a broth on to simmer—a cluster of plump chicken parts and water—and after it cooked for some time, I began adding a few vegetables that had looked appealing and fresh at the market. Sensing her anxiety, I threw in potatoes to contribute a heartier, grounding element. Noting her pallor, I added ginger for extra warmth. And then a few shakes from my collection of bottled condiments—Bragg Liquid Aminos and a touch of rice wine—to achieve a satisfying harmony of sweet, sour, and salty tastes.

When the soup was ready, I poured big bowls for all of us. Steam rose in our faces, turning our cheeks rosy, and as she drank her first spoonful, the new mother visibly softened, as if melting into the heat. Her tense shoulders released, worried brow relaxed, and her body looked more filled and settled. It was a small shift, but an important one: a kind of allowing. The act of eating a meal that had been made with love gave her permission to feel what she was feeling and be in sadness and joy at once. Her most basic needs were met—being fed and being seen—and she could rest and feel safe.

When food is exchanged between friends or loved ones, it creates a powerful sense of connection. Food feeds the cells and fills the senses, and it also nourishes the vulnerable and hidden parts of ourselves that may be crying out for encouragement and comfort. Something as simple as a container of soup, passed from my hands to a baby's father at the hospital elevator, or left in a cooler outside the family home, carries in it ample nutrients and so much more. It is a way to deliver care and love that is received in a woman's innermost core—the perfect, wordless gesture for a quiet, private time.

the postpartum kitchen

Traditionally in China, the postpartum kitchen was the matriarch's domain. Armed with multiple cooking pots and massive ladles, the mother-in-law, auntie, or grandmother would oversee the all-important task of feeding the younger mom and ensuring that no recovery needs got neglected. She wouldn't need to consult a recipe book to do this. The daily menu that she would prepare for this month or more of confinement care would have been handed down from great-grandmother to grandmother, and from grandmother to her. By hearing their stories and watching them at work, the older woman would have absorbed a complex code of feminine knowledge about after-birth care.

She'd know intuitively that pig trotters with ginger and vinegar would purify the blood and alleviate wind and dampness, and she'd serve liver and wine soup to support the circulation. If her young charge looked too pale, she might cluck her tongue and whip up pigeon stew with lily buds to counter extreme fatigue.

And forget about pitchers of water by the bedside table. Though the breastfeeding mother would need to stay well hydrated, plain old water would be considered not just too "cold" (and possibly a health risk if not from a natural spring), but also a lost opportunity for a health perk. Instead, the kitchen mistress would serve endless cups of longan and red date tea for its revitalizing effect, and if she was *really* serious, would insist mom sip ginger wine all day for an extra warming boost. (Yes—wine. This drink's warming property apparently trumped concerns about alcohol content.)

The matriarchs of China knew that the kitchen is where you heal the people you love. Using food as medicine was in their bones, and the ingredients they tossed in the pot weren't added just for their taste: They brought priceless benefits of greater vitality, beauty, and longevity. (The right foods, it was said, would help you live to a hundred, with skin smooth and firm like a ripe plum.)

Furthermore, consuming specialty dishes for certain seasons of your life such as puberty, pregnancy, or old age was pure common sense—as obvious as wearing certain clothes in January and others in July. In this *Tao*, or balanced way, of eating, your diet was chosen to address the body's shifting needs, balance out any extreme states, or replenish any lacks—not just to feed the sudden urge for, say, spaghetti and meatballs.

For the new mother, this meant meals rich in iron to rebuild blood, protein to repair tissues and support hormones, fatty acids to enrich the breast milk, vitamins and antioxidants to speed tissue healing, and therapeutic herbs and spices to counter inflammation or boost milk flow, if needed. She couldn't take a few pre- or postnatal vitamins and consider the job done—her daily meals and drinks had to truly do the job of nourishing and building her up.

Seen through our Western lens, some of *zuo yuezi's* nutritional commandments are extreme: It is said that in Southwest China, a postpartum woman was fed eight to ten eggs a day so baby would get ample cholesterol from her milk for his developing brain. Certainly, eating copious pig kidneys in order to rebuild one's *own* kidney yang, as my own Auntie Ou did for fifty-four days, is not for the faint of heart. It's hard to imagine most contemporary women being able to—or wanting to—stomach such quantities of these high-nutrient foods. (And I'm not convinced it's such a good idea; it is possible to have too much of a good thing.) Yet there is wisdom to reclaim: The way you eat after giving birth can fuel, build, and heal you, and it is often the humblest food that does it best.

I love diving into the tales and customs of traditional eating and healing. There are pearls of wisdom aplenty to be found in the nooks and crannies of this knowledge, and some impressively complex dishes (think: turtle soup) requiring all sorts of tricky ingredients. But when it comes to cooking for new mothers in the here and now, I have extracted the fundamentals from the traditions— the parts of the dishes that capture the essence of the approach—from the all-important "warming" aspect to energy-giving and blood-building properties to lactation support. I borrow a few key items from my aunts' pantries and use them sparingly, alongside everyday fare. In this way, traditions get reinterpreted into something simpler and more aligned with the lifestyles that the women I cook for actually lead—simple dishes that have universal appeal and are accessible to make as well.

It helps that the fundamentals of *zuo yuezi* eating, as for most other post-partum care rituals around the world, fall at the appealingly easy and soft-and-fuzzy end of the cooking spectrum: soups, broths, porridges, steamed and roasted vegetables, stews, and teas—anything that can be poured or heaped into a rounded vessel that will warm your hands and belly. When it comes to filling your cup, it's all about the bowl.

the first forty days food

Cauldrons of soups, pots of fragrant teas, bowls of steaming rice—everything on the table during the first forty days is comfortingly round. How fitting for this closing chapter of the cycle of birth, a time of magnificently curvy body parts and mother cocooning in her nest.

The process of creating these recipes was equally circular. There is nothing linear or logical about the soup-making style of a Chinese auntie. Watching one work in her kitchen is like sitting in a science lab without a textbook. She knows without a word what to cook in order to soothe you—sizing up in a heartbeat whether you're run-down, stressed out, or overly excited. But she won't have the antidote written down in words. "It's in my bones," she'll say or, "Grandmother is whispering in my ear." And forget measuring spoons and weighing scales. The minor details of food prep such as amounts, proportions, and timing are a little flexible.

The recipes that follow share this spirit. They are templates: basic ideas that can be made easily and adapted infinitely, depending on what you have on hand in your kitchen and what you like to eat. This is about sustenance, not gourmet cuisine! You'll find lots of large, one-pot meals that you can eat over several days and that don't require much kitchen know-how to prepare. Almost everything can handle a wildcard ingredient of your choice thrown in, and many can be customized using leftovers from the day before. Enhance or modify these foods according to what appeals in the moment or by playing with some of the tips and suggestions that follow. Once you become familiar with the basic ideas, you might get in the flow completely, and forgo the measuring spoons, too.

Traditional postpartum eating prescribed a significant amount of animal products—meats, bone broths, saturated animal fats, and organ meats, as well as eggs, fish, and, in some cases, dairy. All of these are included here. Moms who eat a primarily plant-based diet may want to try some of these foods for this short duration of time, or they may not. Rest assured, there are plenty of plant-based dishes and drinks shared here that will deliver protein and good fats. Please customize them in the ways you like best, adding any nutrient-dense accents you enjoy (coconut fat, nutritional yeast, bee pollen, and more) wherever you choose. If you choose to use soy-based products, I recommend sticking with tempeh, which is made with fermented soybeans and is less harmful to women's hormones than tofu. Please choose organic tempeh, which will be made from non-GMO soybeans.

If you cook a lot already, or even if you just follow food trends by eating out, you'll find much of what follows feels familiar. Traditional cooking is back in fashion—first it was slow cooking in the spotlight, then it was the rock star rise of bone broths, and now savory rice porridge and oxtail stews are showing up on blogs and at pop-up restaurants worldwide. A new generation is discovering that older, simpler ways of cooking—call it grandmother cooking!—are extremely down to earth. If the kitchen is not your domain, take heart: Chances are good that your friends who do enjoy cooking will find it a breeze to pick up this book and keep you fed.

As to how and when to eat them: *The First Forty Days* is absolutely not a rigid dietary program. Can you imagine wanting to follow a specific regimen with a newborn in your arms? It would feel like the antithesis of the rule-free world you're now living in, where baby eats at all hours of the night and you don't put on shoes for days. And besides, birth and mothering is not a one-size-fits-all experience—every woman has her own way of doing it and her own needs to satisfy. The recipes are loosely organized by style of dish or drink. As you flip through them, take this freedom to heart. Consider the gentle guidelines offered on what foods to embrace and what to avoid, and which dishes might be most suitable for your very early days as a mother. But aside from that, listen to yourself and select dishes and drinks based on what *you* feel your body or mind needs to be comfortable, vital, and calm.

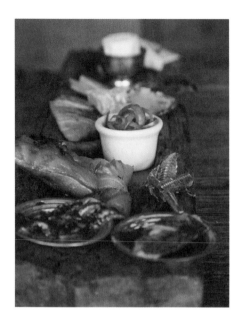

If this "intuitive" way of feeling out what your body wants to eat sounds easier said than done, keep in mind that every physical sensation is magnified after giving birth—from those surges of hunger after breastfeeding to the chills you might feel when you're tired or underfed. Before you eat, take a minute to ask yourself, "Where am I depleted? What do I need to eat right now?" You may find that your food instincts are really awakened, perhaps for the first time.

Of course, you can also just pick your dishes according to what looks really easy to make or what you know you like already—two good enough reasons!

A notable fact in the traditional postpartum protocols is that they all tend to feature a small number of foods served many times. Mom typically consumes the same dishes over and over, keeping things extremely simple and reaping the healing benefits of a few key foods and drinks. This is a huge relief to all involved. You (or your helpers) don't have to cook everything from scratch daily. Make a big pot of soup or stew and eat it for a few meals (try customizing the servings as you go—add a handful of noodles or a whisked-in egg). Then let friends look at this book and make you other things you've never tried. The new mother's mantra is this: *Eating well can mean eating very simply.*

And when the first wave of help subsides and you face the prospect of preparing meals from scratch for yourself, remember: *You can do this.* Putting food on to warm while a baby naps in the next room or washing rice with him strapped on your chest is what women have done for millennia. Whether your heritage is Chinese like mine, or Native American or Irish or Spanish or something else entirely, your ancestors almost certainly cooked simple food with their free hand, and chances are they weren't overly stressed about achieving perfect results. This way of cooking *is* in our bones. We just forgot how natural feeding ourselves can be.

the gentle guidelines

1. THINK SOFT. Postpartum traditions around the world favor food that is soft, soupy, warm, moist, creamy, oily, and fairly mild—with a touch of sweet here and there—for the initial period after birth. If that sounds a little like baby food, it is! After the energetic expenditure of birth and almost ten months of having your abdominal organs pushed into a tighter space, your digestion is considered to be a little slower and weaker than normal, so it's time to eat gently for a while before getting back into high gear. Soupy foods that are already in a smashed-up, semi-liquid, and warm state are optimal, especially in the first week or two. As the warm liquid flows down your throat and into your stomach—that all-important cauldron of digestion that powers your whole body—it meets the warm environment of digestive juices, and it takes less energy for the body to digest and absorb the nutrients. This literally leaves you warmer, with more energy for heating your body and for healing and regenerating. (This is why soup has been mankind's go-to convalescent food since cooking was first invented.) The moistness helps to replenish the liquids lost during birth and counter the dryness in the digestive system that can lead to constipation.

If this food sounds too lightweight for you, consider this: soft, creamy, moist foods can include coconut-milk curries, slow-cooked lentil soup, shredded meat in stock like Cuba's *ropa vieja*, and more. Every culture has its interpretation. Some of the recipes in *The First Forty Days* include accents of Asia like ginger, but there's plenty of room for improvisation if you have favorite ingredients in your pantry.

Consider how a big bowl of food like this spreads warmth through you, as if your belly is glowing like a sun. That's the effect we want to achieve—warming you from the inside out. In addition, foods like beans, rice, and almonds can be soaked first to make them softer and more digestible, or cooked for longer with more liquid to become mushier.

As for which dishes to eat when, the general direction is to start with the foods that are lighter—ginger fried rice is one of the first foods eaten after birth in China, and *miyeokguk* (seaweed soup) is brought to hospitals in Korea—and work up to heavier stews and denser dishes as your digestive fire gets stronger. Nothing is set in stone. Let your body be your guide: If you feel tired and chilly after a bigger, heavier meal, it could be a sign that this particular combination of ingredients is too taxing right now.

NOTE: *The recipes include few wheat or gluten-containing products, mainly because these things have not traditionally been used in the healing cuisines that inspire me. That does not mean you need to take a gluten-free stance; adapt the recipes as you like, and continue eating what your body is used to. This is not the time to make radical alterations.*

2. NIX THE COLD. Since the goal is to keep your body warm, consuming cold foods and icy drinks is one of the few actual no-nos. Eastern traditions eschew frigid foods and iced water almost all the time—not just postpartum—because consuming them is like throwing cold water on the digestive fire. They say it literally slows down or "stagnates" digestion, forcing your stomach and spleen to work unnecessarily hard, and even counsel that eating food straight from the refrigerator is stressful—and unnatural. (Consider how fridges didn't even exist in most households until a few generations ago.) Be sure to set out foods and drinks that won't be heated for at least half an hour before consuming, so they can get to room temperature.

For a new mother, this is key because cold in the abdominal region can stagnate the circulation of blood necessary for returning the womb and reproductive system to a healthy, nonpregnant state. This may sound like an old wives' tale, but many women will notice the effect of eating ice cream during their menstrual periods: It causes a coagulation of blood flow and exacerbates cramping. The stagnating impact of coldness is something you can actually track.

In addition to steering clear of foods that are physically cold to touch, new mothers are advised to avoid food with cooling properties. This is a little subtler. It means foods that, after digestion and absorption, cool the body. Watermelons, cucumbers, and radishes are obvious contenders, and, in fact, all raw vegetables and fruits are seen to be cooling, as well as cold dairy foods like milk and yogurt.

Interestingly, Ayurveda explains that eating *crunchy* foods will exacerbate the excess *vata* or air in the new mother's system, which disrupts digestion and causes airy, anxious mental states. Combine these two ideas, and it means that eating a big bowl of ice cream and pretzels, or even chilled crudités, soon after birth is the equivalent of running outside in a windstorm wearing a tank top, whereas spooning up some warm rice congee is like sinking into a hot tub with fluffy towels all around. The recipes here will help you by simply omitting the primary cooling-food culprits.

But what if you get a craving for a few carrots or a fresh salad? By all means, eat it and enjoy it. Just be moderate and above all, don't skew your diet toward raw. Throw your fresh spinach in a blender, if you like, to make a Joyful Green Smoothie (page 186). This is served at room temperature and includes some healthy fats that counter the "cold" vegetable with warmth. And if the vanilla ice cream is just too tempting to resist, have it—only occasionally, please—in between meals, so your inner fire gets a chance to flare back up before the main course is served. Notice if you feel much colder than normal after consuming it. The kinder way to satisfy this urge would be with a Spiced Vanilla Egg Custard (page 202)—similar ingredients, better temperature!

3 . LOVE YOUR FATS. Postpartum is the time to kindle a love affair with good fats in your food and ensure you consume them steadily. Traditionally, the postpartum mother's diet has always included meals rich in saturated fats and key omega fatty acids (such as arachidonic acid and DHEA) that are essential for her baby's nervous system development. These things come from animal fats, quality eggs, oily fish (and extractions like cod liver oil) and, studies have shown, they quantifiably enrich the breast milk, helping baby's brain grow and thrive.

These fats also are critical for you to thrive. Fats are the premium-grade gas in your tank that, calorie for calorie, gives you more energy than any other food source. Eating a diet filled with good fats—your choice of grass- and pasture-raised meat and butter, oily cold-water fish like sardines, and raw plant fats and oils like coconut, olive, walnut, sesame, and avocado—is critical postpartum. It will boost your metabolism so your body will be able to gradually get to the healthy weight that's right for you over the months to come. (Research shows that protein from pasture-fed animals helps build a healthy immune system and saturated fat helps supply the body with usable energy that doesn't store on the body as fat. Promise!) It will enhance circulation so you are warm from the inside out; it will help to balance hormones, supporting your mood, and help your brain function, keeping you confident and clear. And it will lubricate your intestines, helping to keep digestion moving and keeping you comfortable.

Keep healthy fats in mind as you fill each bowl, cup, or glass. You'll find a spectrum of ways to include them in the recipes here—from adding bacon to a pork broth to stirring raw butter into warm drinks—and you can customize recipes as you like. If you already cook with good-quality lard—a fabulous saturated fat—use it for cooking any of the stews. If dairy digests well for you, stir soft and creamy goat cheese into any hot dish. Above all, remember: Should you feel the chills, stir rich coconut milk into a mug of hot tea, or have some nut butter from the jar—whatever will quickly get some fat into your system. Fats are the surefire way to stoke your inner furnace.

4. OBSERVE HOW YOUR FOOD (MIGHT) AFFECT YOUR BABY, but don't obsess about it. Every culture from East to West labels certain foods off-limits for a breastfeeding mother: specific items that can aggravate baby by causing gas in her tiny belly after she drinks your milk. These range from large beans and legumes to cruciferous vegetables (cauliflower, cabbage, brussels sprouts, kale, collards) and cold pasteurized milk to fermented foods like sauerkraut, and more.

After consuming one of the taboo foods, your baby *may* emit pained cries—which is excruciating for the worried mother, too—and have a taut belly. This is a sign of gas and certainly a cue to avoid that food. But there may be no effect at all, especially if you typically tolerate these foods just fine. No book or healer can tell you more than your own body can. So, rather than following strict rules, use gentle recipes, designed to be low in gas-forming compounds, and focus on baby and notice how he reacts after certain meals. And refrain from becoming neurotic about the gas issue—having guilt about what you innocently ate for dinner will only add stress. The truth is that newborns do cry a fair amount and often do have digestive growing pains as they get used to life outside the womb. The crying may not be all mom's fault! (If painful gas is an issue, serving baby small amounts of organic gripe water, made from digestive herbs, is often extremely helpful—it can be found at most health food stores—as is very gentle tummy massage in a clockwise circle with a bit of sesame or olive oil, and ask your doctor about baby probiotics—current research supports their efficacy in helping baby's digestion.)

The recipes here fold in the anti-gas secrets of the ages by using small and digestible beans (soaking them for a few hours before cooking helps to make them less gassy); by choosing warm or hot milk over cold; nut milks instead of dairy if your body finds cow's milk irritating; and spices and herbs like ginger, fennel, and chamomile that are prized for their ability to balance out gas. Tougher greens like kale should be well cooked (and possibly avoided for the first two weeks or more, while your newborn's system is especially fresh. If in doubt, substitute spinach). But remember, the fine workings of the digestive system are not fully predictable, so my suggestion in regard to gas is relax, observe, and adapt as you go.

Of course, if something you eat gives *you* palpable gas, steer clear for a while. That's a no-brainer.

5. DRINK UP. You need to replenish liquids lost in birth and help your body create a whole *new* kind of liquid food: breast milk. Keep jugs of room temperature water near your bed and nursing chair and drink a glass at every feeding. Sipping warm water is even better—it's customary in Asia as it delivers free warmth. You don't have to force down gallons more H_2O than normal; just set yourself up to keep sipping and stay hydrated, remembering the 8x8 equation (8 glasses, 8 ounces/240 ml each). But also turn to the recipes. Bone broth is a brilliant, savory drink that confers energy without taxing the digestive system, because it hydrates you and lubricates your intestines. The herbal tea recipes may also be drunk in quantity; fill up your water bottle with warm or room temperature Red Dates and Goji Tea or Nettle and Fennel Tea (page 207) and sip those as you would water.

From an Ayurvedic perspective, drinking hot water throughout the day is essential after birth. It gives you free heat; it is nurturing and soothing, and when sipped between meals, it calms that burning hunger from stomach acid that makes you reach impulsively for a packaged snack instead of preparing a good plate. Hot water also helps you make better decisions, because it soothes your gut. The best decisions are gut decisions—and you need those now more than ever.

—VASU DUDAKIA, AYURVEDIC PRACTITIONER, LOS ANGELES, CA

6. LET YOUR VILLAGE COOK. Good news: The recipes for the Gateway can be made by committee. Delegate the duties according to people's skill sets. The person who is a seasoned cook can make you a dish from scratch, or pull out a bag of frozen broth, locate the necessary ingredients in your nicely organized postpartum pantry, and get a soup or stew on to simmer; a rookie in the kitchen can wash and prep vegetables for steaming, blitz a smoothie, or just put out a snack. Appeal to the hunter-gatherer sides of some of the men in your village and give them your small but focused shopping list of fresh items that you need. And remember, anyone can do the dishes and mop the floor. You just have to ask.

VICE OR NICE?
COFFEE, WINE, AND MORE

You probably dramatically—or completely—reduced your caffeine intake during pregnancy. So is it safe to consume a latte now? Traces of caffeine do make it into breast milk and the truth is it is harder for a newborn, with his tender "fourth trimester" body, to metabolize and excrete it than it is for an older infant, so it could stimulate his nervous system. (It might also impact you: Caffeine inhibits the absorption of iron, so do not consume it alongside iron-rich foods.) If consumed in amounts of 3 cups (750 ml) or more a day, baby will likely be very aggravated—not a very welcoming entry to the world outside the womb.

To be on the safe side, consider if you can go without caffeine for the first forty days and accept any blurriness as a new (and temporary) state of being. Or, will decaf coffee, with its traces of caffeine, actually give you enough of a lift? There are lots of good coffee substitutes on the market, like Teeccino and other chicory blends. Ceremonial Hot Chocolate (page 216) or Chocolate Hazelnut Milk (page 183) might surprise you with cacao's uplifting effect. Nettle Infusion (page 208) subtly energizes the body in a sustained way and, strange as it may sound, broths of all kind drunk from a mug in the morning are quite grounding and energizing. I love drinking a mug of Fish Broth (page 132) first thing.

If the urge for caffeine is unstoppable, there are always the obvious coffee stand-ins: Green tea is much less caffeinated and black tea has a slightly higher quantity than green. And a single espresso contains considerably less caffeine than a tall cup of drip-brewed coffee. Don't become caught up in hard and rigid rules, but stay connected to your baby, watch for signs, and be gentle on the both of you.

Perhaps most important, if you do drink a little coffee, please choose organic. Conventionally grown coffee beans have some of the highest amounts of pesticides of any crop. Plus, the decaffeination process typically uses chemical solvents to extract the caffeine from the bean, so an organic brand, or one that you can verify uses a water-based extraction process, is safer for baby and you.

Evening brings with it another conundrum: Can mom sink into a moment of tranquility with a glass of Cabernet? Traditionalists did serve ginger wine after all, and in some cultures, beer is actually taken to stimulate prolactin levels and boost milk production. (It's an effect of the barley, however, not the alcohol.) Most experts agree that moderate consumption of beer or wine by a breastfeeding mother (think: an occasional small glass) will not adversely affect baby. That said, during the Gateway, *everything is magnified*. You are easing a newborn into the world and his liver is still immature. If you are going to imbibe a bit, have it with a meal and try to let your body metabolize the alcohol before you nurse—about two to three hours for a glass of wine or beer (the ethanol in breast milk reduces as the blood alcohol levels decrease). If your breasts engorge uncomfortably in this time, you might hand express or pump the milk and discard it. (Hard alcohol, as you might imagine, should be completely avoided.) Try joining the celebration with a martini glass filled with Ginger Lemonade Switchel (page 73)—you'll get a probiotic benefit instead of booze.

what to eat and when to eat it

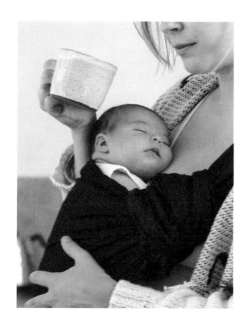

Forget breakfast, lunch, and dinner, if you like. Since regular scheduling goes out the window with a newborn, don't be beholden to typical mealtimes or portion sizes. *Eat to feed your need*, not the time of day. If you're awake and hungry at 3 A.M., warm up a big mug of nut milk or a bowl of congee. If you've been up for ages at 7 A.M., a bowl of soup might be just the ticket. (In Asia, soup and chicken congee are considered excellent breakfasts.) Be sure to consume some protein in the morning to get your day of caretaking—and milk production—off to a solid start, and please include substantial dishes in the mix as you go. Lighter eating works well for the first few days, but after that, it's important for the new mother to take in plenty of protein, fats, and slow-releasing carbohydrates—*do not* subsist on broth and steamed greens alone! Use the smoothies, nut milks, and snacks at any time to keep your energy intake up. Above all, keep nourishing yourself with steady, consistent sustenance and, if eating is not the first thing on your mind, ask others to help you stay well fed.

One caveat: In the early days of parenting, it's fine to let family dinner time fall by the wayside. Your partner will likely need heartier food than you do, and you may find yourself eating different foods at different times. But if you have been the primary cook in the home, it will leave a gap in the food supply, so now's the time to ensure that your helping hands team is delivering meals so that everyone stays fed. As time goes by and you get into your groove a little more, I recommend that you share a meal a day with your partner, perhaps creating a cozy dinner as baby snuggles up next to you on the sofa (she can't crawl or roll over yet!). Eating is an act of togetherness that anchors the family—it is a moment to connect.

the postpartum pantry

What follows are the foods that I suggest having on hand for the first forty days. I list the staple ingredients that are most commonly used in the recipes, plus a few things that you might want to nibble on at random, and some specialty items that you can get by without—but that I hope you'll feel inspired to try. They are all simple, whole foods. They include dried and nonperishable goods that should be stored in the cupboard or pantry (if you have one), fresh items to keep in the fridge that can be replenished every week or so, and a few items for the freezer.

You'll see that there are lots of options suggested, so that you can use things you already like (or already have). You don't need to do a complete kitchen makeover to make the dishes here. It's important to let your pantry take shape according to what you already like to eat and keep things easy and familiar. There are plenty of new ideas and ingredients to try in the recipe section if you like, but it can all be anchored in the foods you already know how to make and enjoy.

Most of these ingredients can be purchased at grocery stores, many can be found at healthier stores like Whole Foods or co-ops, a smattering require specialty stores or websites, and much of the shopping could even be consolidated through a bulk order online, so your provisions get shipped to your door (see "Pantry Resources," page 124). Having a good spectrum of the staple ingredients and some of the specialty ingredients will put you in good stead for eating well in the days and weeks to come. Whether your partner or a helping-hand friend is doing the cooking in your kitchen, or you are doing much of it yourself, if your pantry is stocked and organized with these very practical and functional whole-food ingredients, there will be plenty of satisfying things you can make.

As for questions of quality: Purchasing all organic and locally produced foods is a worthy ideal, but with all the costs of having a baby, that might be unrealistic for you. Don't stress about perfecting your system today. Do the best your resources—both financial and time—will allow. These nourishing foods will hopefully become staples of your family meals for years to come. You can gradually upgrade your sources as you find the most affordable and healthiest options near you. I include "What to Look For" info to help you pick the best option when you do have the luxury of choice.

THE FIRST FORTY DAYS MEALS:
A CHEAT SHEET

SIMPLE FIRST FOODS: particularly suited to postdelivery (and great anytime thereafter as well)

- Ginger Fried Rice
- Chicken, Red Dates & Ginger Soup
- Postpartum Egg-Drop Soup with Liver & Greens
- C-Recovery Vegetable Stew
- White Rice Congee and variations
- Mother's Bowl featuring soft scrambled eggs, avocado, cooked grains

HEARTIER MEALS: for a stronger appetite and meals shared with your partner; cooked in advance and frozen in portions, or ask members of your "meal train" to make them for you

- Hearty Sausage Stew
- Oxtail Stew
- C-Recovery Vegetable Stew

LACTATION AIDS: to support let down and flow

- Fish, Papaya & Peanut Soup
- Seaweed Soup
- Oats & Chia Congee
- Nettle & Fennel Tea
- Cumin & Fenugreek Tea
- Herb Infusions (various)

QUICK HITS: even a rookie in the kitchen can make these for you

- PB & J Smoothie
- Cashew & Chia Milk
- Ceremonial Hot Chocolate
- Pink Cranberry Porridge
- Oats & Chia Congee

SURVIVAL SNACKS: especially the 1 + 1 ingredient pairings

- Mother's Bowls
- Ginger Fried Rice

KID-FRIENDLY DISHES: any other children in the home will especially enjoy these

- Sweet Rice Congee with Black Sesame Paste
- Mexican Bowl
- Peanut Butter & Honey Rice Crispy Treats
- Chocolate Mousse
- Gooey Chocolate Brownies
- Ginger Fried Rice (if it's not obvious by now, this one's a staple—make sure to give it a try!)

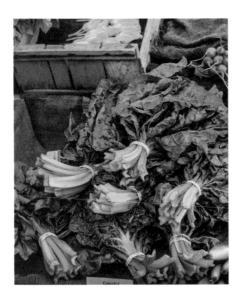

VEGETABLES

Put vegetables and fruits on a weekly shopping list and replenish as necessary.

Onions (yellow) and garlic: These are used frequently in soups. Shallots and green (or spring) onions are also used fairly frequently.

Ginger: Keep a big knob on hand, stored in a plastic bag in the fridge. (See also "Specialty Items," page 120.) Note: Ginger can increase blood flow. If you notice that your postpartum bleeding has intensified after consuming dishes that include ginger, avoid those recipes for two weeks (when postpartum bleeding slows significantly) or omit it from the recipe.

Greens: Buy a variety for soups, bowls, and smoothies. Pick any greens that are fresh, appealing, and local, if possible. Examples: spinach, kale, Swiss chard, collard greens, and spicy greens like mizuna and arugula. Dandelion, nettles, and turnip greens are also fair game. It's also fine to have frozen spinach in the freezer as a backup!

Root vegetables: Keep a stash of your favorites for roasting. This can include sweet potatoes and/or white potatoes, yams and/or Japanese white or purple sweet potatoes, and winter squash (your choice of kabocha, acorn, butternut, delicata). Potatoes, carrots, and parsnips are also used in some of the recipes and can be added to bulk out others.

Mushrooms: A nutritional boon that also boost immunity and increase vitamin D levels. Though fresh shiitake are slightly pricey, they can be worth the splurge and are used several times in the recipes. A handful of plain white and button varieties can also work wonderfully.

Other seasonal vegetables: Think turnips, radishes, rutabaga, peas, green beans, nettles, and celery root. Almost any other vegetables that friends might bring over can be cooked into bowls, stews, and soups. Just be moderate in consumption of cruciferous vegetables (cauliflower, brussels sprouts, broccoli, bok choy, cabbage) and watch if they irritate baby's digestion.

Embrace these foods	Minimize or avoid these foods
Soups, stews, broths, stewed fruits	Salads, raw vegetables
Warm cooked grains	Crunchy crackers, chips
Chicken, slow-cooked lamb, beef/bison	Heavy meat, like steaks, organ meats
Custards, steamed puddings	Ice cream, sorbet, gelato
Warm milk, soft goat cheese, unsweetened whole-milk yogurt, hard cheese (use in moderation)	Sweetened skim yogurt, sweetened kefir
Fish, including oily fish, sea vegetables (sardines, mackerel, herring)	
Avocados, coconut, olives (whole foods or oils)	Processed and refined cooking oils (canola, sunflower)
Seed, nut oils (sesame, hemp oils)	
Fat stirred into everything (grass-fed butter, coconut oil, coconut milk, ghee)	
Warming ginger, cinnamon, cumin, turmeric	
Herbal teas and infusions	Strong caffeine, coffee
Kombucha and other naturally fermented non-alcoholic beverages	Wine and beer (use in moderation), avoid liquor

Jars of store-bought kimchee and/or sauerkraut: Use both on congee and Mother's Bowls to add flavor, boost nutrition, aid digestion and elimination, and get immune-boosting probiotics in your diet. The unpasteurized kind is best, with enzymes and probiotics still intact.

FRUITS

Fresh or frozen berries, and bananas, for smoothies. Try to have several avocados in stock at all times, a papaya if you choose to make Fish, Papaya & Peanut Soup (page 178), and tomatoes—a fruit!—can be fresh, but canned are fine, too. Any other seasonal fruit you love, like apples and pears, can be easily simmered with water plus a little ginger to make delicious servings of warm, stewed fruit.

What to look for: I prefer fresh and local fruits and vegetables over organic produce that has been shipped from far away, losing nutritional content in transit. Local (farmers' market) produce is often pesticide-free even when not "certified organic." The musts for buying organic are strawberries and mushrooms, due to their very thin skins, and corn if you use it, because of risk factors from eating GMO crops.

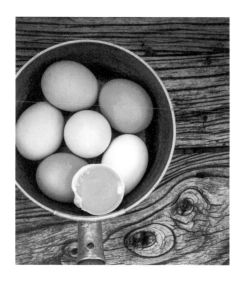

EGGS, MEAT, AND FISH

Have your choices of the following in the fridge, freezer, or pantry. Replenish as necessary.

Eggs: Treat yourself to pasture-raised eggs to get the maximum nutritional bonus. Their yolks should be bright orange. Eggs from local sources (farmer's markets or small farms) usually trump organic-labeled eggs in the grocery store. These "organic" eggs may be from chickens that were kept in cages and fed an all-grain diet, which isn't ideal. Free-range and omnivorous chickens (who have eaten insects and such) and their eggs are best.

Meat: Chicken, beef, lamb, and pork are all used here, but you can easily adapt things with other types like turkey, bison, duck, or even wild-caught game like venison. Recipes use whole chickens or chicken parts, ground red meat or sliced flank, and sausages.

Fresh or frozen whole fish or fillets: Used in Fish Broth (page 132); Fish, Papaya & Peanut Soup (page 178); and to serve cooked in Mother's Bowls (page 167). Check Food and Water Watch online to see which fresh fish is sustainable where you live and if the kinds you see in the market are on the "safe" list, as it often changes. It's a wonderful resource. Canned wild salmon, sardines, mackerel, and herring are excellent provisions for the pantry and readily available at most grocery stores. The Wild Planet brand is one of my favorites.

Bones: For broth, made in advance or at any time during first forty days. In addition to typical beef, chicken, or pork "soup bones," seek out knuckle and marrow bones, pig's feet (trotters), and chicken feet when you can. I highly recommend getting these items from pastured animals that have been raised outside, not factory-farmed or grain-fed animals—if your grocery does not have these, farmer's markets and local ranches and farms often do, at great prices. Adding these parts to your broth when possible gives it a superb nutritional boost, with lots of healing gelatin.

What to look for: Grass-fed and pasture-raised meats, eggs, and dairy will give a healthier fatty-acid profile than grain-fed ones, meaning a better balance of omega-3 to omega-6, and have more essential vitamins. Buying from a local farm that sells meat is often good as they usually have organic practices, even if they don't pay the extra fee to use the label "certified organic." I'd choose grass-fed or pastured meat without the "organic" stamp over certified-organic meat that has been grain-fed and may not have been raised in humane ways.

DRIED FRUIT, NUTS, AND SEEDS

Dried Fruit: Any and all of your choice. Prunes can be good for encouraging your elimination; Turkish figs, used in one of the granola recipes, are delicious and may satisfy a craving for sweets—and the seeds are mild laxatives, which addresses the constipation that can occur after birth. Unsulphured and unsweetened dried fruit is best, if you can get it.

Nuts: Almonds, cashews, macadamia, and hazelnuts are used in the recipes, but don't forget walnuts, pecans, and pistachios, if you like them. Raw or dry-roasted nuts are best. If you can, avoid the oil roasted and salted ones. You can always add your own salt later if you like.

Seeds: Chia, flax, hemp, sunflower, and white and black sesame seeds (see also "Specialty Items," page 120) are used in smoothies and as toppings in the bowls.

BEANS AND GRAINS

Beans: Adzuki beans are the easiest beans to digest, small, and non–gas forming. They're used in congees, stews, and bowls. Garbanzos (chickpeas) are thrown into stews, but other beans of your choice (white, black, kidney, pinto) can be added, too. Canned beans are most convenient but bulk-bought dried beans are very economical choices for a family, if you are familiar with preparing them.

Lentils: Red, green, black—and don't forget about the tinier varieties, like Le Puy, that cook faster.

Rice: It's always helpful to have a variety on hand. White and sticky (also called glutinous) rices are most often used in congees, and brown, basmati, black, and wild rice are other options for bowls and sides. Puffed (hard) rice is used in granola and rice crispy treats or as a simple gluten-free breakfast cereal (sort of like Rice Krispies).

Oats: Recipes in this book use steel-cut oats and regular rolled oats, organic if possible. They're good to have on hand for granola, pancakes, oatmeal, congees, even comforting cookies. Something that lasts in the pantry and is super grounding and warming, oats are a good source of iron and may help produce more breast milk. They are also available in gluten-free versions.

Other whole grains of your choice can include gluten-containing ones such as barley, which is used in a lactation tea, and non-gluten grains like quinoa, millet, amaranth, and buckwheat (not actually a grain, but a delicious and hearty grain-like food).

Noodles: Any type. This could be thin Asian-style noodles made of rice, soba (buckwheat), or eggs, or thicker ones made of wheat, corn, and even bean, and/or pasta made with the same ingredients. They are great and quick additions to broths, soups, and stews. If you're using gluten-free noodles and other packaged goods, watch out for xanthum gum (which can upset your stomach; many people are sensitive to it) and try to choose non-GMO brands whenever possible.

Polenta: A great and easy addition to stews and bowls. If you buy it already cooked (Trader Joe's has logs of precooked organic polenta), you can slice it into rounds and fry it for a hearty side or "bread-like" snack in minutes.

What to look for: I like to use organic grains whenever possible, to get the extra nutrition that has been measured in them and to avoid chemical exposure. This is especially important with wheat products as wheat crops are often sprayed multiple times before harvesting and treated during processing, and those chemicals have been linked to autism and neurological problems in children.

DAIRY PRODUCTS AND ALTERNATIVES

Milk, yogurt, cream, kefir, and cheese: These typically cooling foods are not used a lot in *The First Forty Days* recipes, but if you like and enjoy them, by all means have them on hand. Interestingly, goat milk is a warming food in Chinese medicine (it is much easier to digest than cow's milk). Raw dairy is a true super food, if you have access to it. Organic dairy is well worth the cost to minimize your and baby's exposure to toxins. Consume dairy foods warm when possible and use them in moderation; if baby seems to have digestive distress after you've eaten or drunk lots of dairy, consider backing off.

Grass-fed butter: An amazing postpartum kitchen staple. In one small block of buttercup-yellow fat, you get loads more fat-soluble vitamins than in regular butter (A, E, and D, and the equally essential vitamin K) and crucial micronutrients like those all-important fatty acids for baby's development. Lavishing grass-fed butter onto your cooked greens will help you absorb their vitamins better, and, if you cook meat in it, it helps you digest the protein better. What's not to love? Start smearing butter onto your steaming grains, root vegetables, and greens—or even stirring it into your Ceremonial Hot Chocolate (page 216) or decaf coffee.

Coconut milk: Coconut is another traditional warming food—wonderfully rich in fat! I like using light coconut milk because it is cut with water and is easier to use in smoothies than full-fat coconut milk (which you can of course cut with water yourself). Try to buy it without xanthum gum or sugar. Trader Joe's light coconut milk is sold in BPA-free cans and So Delicious has it in large milk-type containers at most health food stores. When using the canned versions, even the light ones, you may need to thin it with a bit more water as it's thicker than the carton milk.

Almond, hemp, hazelnut, oat, and other nondairy milks: Consider having a few boxes on hand for smoothies and to drink straight when you can't make fresh nut milks. Try to buy a brand without xanthum gum or sweeteners.

MORE PANTRY ITEMS

Nut and seed butters: Almond butter, peanut butter (look for non-GMO and unsweetened), sunflower seed butter or any other nut butter out there, like cashew or walnut, are perfect for snacks, smoothies, and treats. When you need a quick (and quiet) hit of food, peanut or almond butter right out of the jar is comforting and filling. Coconut Manna, sold in jars, is a super-healthy way to treat your body to saturated fat.

Bone broth or stock: When you don't have homemade broth on hand, boxes of vegetable, chicken, and beef broth are a decent substitute. Look for organic and sugar-free kinds. Frozen bone broth can also be ordered in bulk from artisanal producers. Though pricey, this is the real deal and perfect for adding to a wish list.

Canned tomatoes and tomato paste: Fresh is always preferred but use organic cans or tubes of tomatoes and paste in the winter months when it's not fresh.

Organic popcorn: A favorite DIY snack, popcorn has become even tastier and more digestible thanks to the new "heirloom popcorn" varieties now available. At the very least, buy organic (non-GMO) popcorn.

Shredded coconut: Used in sweet recipes, granola, and as a fun add-in to smoothies, desserts, and sweet congees.

Cacao or cocoa powder: For nut milks, smoothies, Ceremonial Hot Chocolate (page 216), mousse, brownies, and granola. Cacao powder is the raw, unprocessed form, with more essential nutrients like magnesium than cocoa.

Cacao nibs: An optional ingredient that is a superb addition to cookies, sweets, smoothies, sweet congee, and even hot tea.

Boxed coconut water: This optional pantry ingredient is nature's sports drink, sweet and replenishing.

Pure vanilla extract: This sweet and fragrant flavoring is so functional; use it to enhance smoothies, sweets, nut milks, cocoas, and teas. Available in traditional alcohol extract form or in glycerin (alcohol-free). Avoid imitation vanilla or ones with sugar.

Black or oolong tea: For drinking in moderation and for making Pickled Congee with Tea Eggs and Pickles (page 159).

Nutritional yeast: This natural seasoning, beloved by vegans in particular, can be sprinkled on lots of dishes to add a satisfying "umami" taste (a cheesy, meaty, savory flavor) and loads of B vitamins, which help your body extract energy from food and help replenish red blood cells.

SWEETENERS

Include a couple of these healthier options in your pantry to flavor sweets and teas.

Honey: Try to use raw honey (available at health food stores or farmer's markets). Since it hasn't been heated, it retains amazing health benefits, intact enzymes and minerals, and proteins. If it comes from a local source, it's an antidote for seasonal allergies where you live as well.

Maple syrup: The real kind, not the corn-syrup blend.

Coconut sugar: A delicious alternative to brown sugar with some good trace minerals, comes in sap or granule form. Especially handy if you don't use honey or maple syrup.

Stevia: It can be handy to have a pack of this noncaloric powdered herb to sweeten things without refined sugar.

OILS AND VINEGARS

A selection of oils infuse your diet with good fat and vinegars, and create great flavors in all kinds of dishes. In the recipes, I list "cooking oil" as an ingredient, which refers to your choice of a high-heat-tolerant oil—coconut, avocado, or lard. Likewise, soy sauce has alternative options depending on your preference and dietary needs. As you get familiar with your oils and flavorings, you can create a harmony of sweet, sour, and salty tastes by using the same few staples. Every traditional kitchen has a cluster of these bottles next to the stove; pick a few and use throughout the recipes.

Sesame oil: A time-honored healing food, sesame oil is used for cooking and can also be used for massage—for mother and baby. Pick organic, expeller-pressed, or unrefined oil.

Avocado oil: Formerly a specialty item, this oil is now found abundantly and is a great cooking oil, as any saturated fat is, since it's stable at high temperatures. (In baking, it can also be a great replacement for coconut oil, which solidifies in the jar and can be hard to remove.)

Coconut oil: Consider acquiring a large jar of this fantastic saturated fat. High in essential omega-3s, including lauric acid, a rare fatty-acid that is also found in breast milk, coconut oil is great for high-heat cooking, can be spooned onto steamed greens or cooked grains, and is a great moisturizing and massage oil for mom's and baby's skin. Refined cooking oil is odorless, so it won't give such a "coconut" flavor to your cooking.

Soy sauce, wheat-free tamari, (soy-free) Bragg Liquid Aminos, nama shoyu (raw soy sauce), or coconut amino acids: Lots of great options and it's your choice. A small amount of these fermented soy (or soy-tasting) condiments add a lot of tangy, salty flavor to soups. You can use them instead of (or in addition to) sea salt.

Vinegar: Apple cider and balsamic vinegars are the options most often used in the recipes. Chinese sweetened black vinegar is also used (see also "Specialty Items," page 120).

Miso: This fermented soybean paste comes from Japanese cuisine and adds a satisfyingly salty, savory flavor when stirred into soups and grains or used as a dip (see "Snacks," page 188). There are several varieties—yellow miso has the mildest flavor. Keep miso in the fridge.

SPICES AND HERBS

Chances are you have a spectrum of these ingredients already. These are the most often-used ones, but expand your collection as you like or as your curiosity dictates.

Himalayan (pink) or Celtic (gray) sea salt: Salt is important for hydration and circulation. Choose a colored salt, not a plain white one, for a rainbow of minerals. Keep in mind that if the gray Celtic sea salt is still slightly moist, which is often the case at health food stores, it's packed with even more minerals!

Ginger: Dried ginger is a good backup when your fresh ginger has run out.

Turmeric: Fresh is great if you can find it, but always have turmeric powder on hand as a backup.

Cinnamon: Ground cinnamon is used in granola and sweets, and sticks are used in teas and soups to add a pleasant, sweet twist without sugar. (The sticks can be ground in a clean coffee grinder, too.)

Fennel seeds: A primary ingredient for lactation tea. Fenugreek and cumin seeds are also used for tea.

Chili or cayenne powder: These warming spices boost circulation and provide heat. They also regulate blood sugar levels and help sluggish metabolisms; the heat raises body temperature, and the body's natural regulating process burns more calories to cool you down.

Cumin: Ground cumin for vegetable soups, and cumin seeds in tea. (The seeds can be ground in a clean coffee grinder, too.)

Herbs for broth: Fresh thyme, oregano, marjoram, rosemary, savory, and basil. You don't necessarily need all of them; one or two to start with is fine.

Herbs for teas and infusions: Choose a few herbs from the "Tea and Infusions" section (page 206) to start, going with what calls to you. Nettle and raspberry leaf are two of the most commonly used by new mothers, along with chamomile and lavender to aid relaxation and sleep. Red clover, goat's rue, blessed thistle and motherwort are other options. See "Pantry Resources" (page 124) for a high-quality organic source.

SPECIALTY ITEMS

These traditional food items may be new to you, but they are lots of fun to use. They will infuse your food with flavor, color, and healing benefits, so I encourage you to get some of them into your pantry—or ask for the pricier ones, marked with a **$** sign, as gifts! See "Pantry Resources" (page 124) for information on where to buy.

Ginger: Though it's as common as corn in American stores these days, ginger is worth a mention as a specialty item. One of the most important ingredients in the traditional *zuo yuezi* pantry, ginger is a medicinal food with exceptional warming properties. It is used in several teas and dishes here. If you buy organic, you won't need to peel it, just wash it first. I recommend really getting to know the gingerroot in your hand—hold it for a few minutes and see how it feels. Simple ginger should get treated with reverence! As mentioned in the vegetables section, ginger can also increase bleeding, so pay attention to your blood flow as you experiment with the recipes. If you experience an uncomfortable surge in bleeding, avoid ginger for two weeks, or until your bleeding notably slows.

Chinese red dates: Also known as jujubes, these dried fruits are classic postpartum fare in China, used as a warming ingredient to help boost circulation while conferring good vitamins and antioxidants. They also have a relaxing effect. Look for unsulphured dates.

Goji berries ($): Used in combination with red dates in Chicken, Red Dates & Ginger Soup (page 138) as well as a classic postpartum tea, goji berries are famous kidney tonics in Chinese medicine—making them terrific for reproductive health.

Dried and medicinal mushrooms ($): Though dried mushrooms are not cheap, they last for ages and add wonderful flavor to soups, stews, and other dishes. Shiitake are used in these recipes, plus the more medicinal reishi mushroom as an optional add-in. Reishi is a legendary adaptogenic herb in Chinese medicine that boosts all systems of the body. Known as the "mushroom of immortality," it is a great entry-level healing fungus that's fairly easy to acquire.

Seaweed: This plant vegetable has historically been consumed postpartum to help the new mom rebuild depleted minerals. You can use one or more types of seaweed in your daily cooking. Strips of kombu cooked in water create Japanese-style dashi or broth; when added to a pot of beans, kombu helps to reduce their gassiness. Scatter tasty dulse flakes into anything you like for a salty tang and a nutrient-dense profile that aids metabolism and thyroid function (it's high in calcium and fiber). And play with sheets of nori—the sushi-roll wrapper. Wrap balls of rice or pieces of fish or avocado in it for a one-hand snack. Bonus: Nori is high in protein and iron. Wakame, arame, and hijiki seaweed can also be used in Seaweed Soup (page 147).

Black sesame seeds: A classic Chinese ingredient famed for its age-defying properties, black sesame is also considered a lactation aid and a remedy for constipation. Its B vitamins and iron help replenish physical depletions—perhaps this is why older Chinese women swear that black sesame seeds will give you glossy, shiny hair. Add them to smoothies and sprinkle them in savory and sweet dishes for extra texture and crunch.

Black vinegar: A famed cure-all in Chinese kitchens, black vinegar is a traditional warming ingredient that boosts blood circulation—especially when it is combined with ginger—and helps with indigestion and constipation. It contains lots of essential amino acids for bodily repair and tissue growth, and, most important, it adds a satisfying tang of flavor to soups and stews.

Organ meats: A revered power food in traditional kitchens worldwide, organ meats like liver and kidney are included here in small doses. Please get them from grass-fed and pastured animals. Chicken and duck liver has the mildest taste, with calf's liver the next mildest.

Great Lakes gelatin ($): This high-grade, powdered gelatin from grass-fed animals is a health supplement that confers many of the amazing benefits of bone broths in a very handy and multifunctional form. It's made of the amino acids glycine and proline, which support skin, hair, and nail growth as well as immune system and weight management—all things that you can use help with after creating and birthing a child! Just like the gelatin you may have used to make cheesecake, this flavorless product thickens into a gel-like texture when stirred into liquid. It is used in the Spiced Vanilla Egg Custard recipe (page 202) and can be stirred into warm cocoa and teas as a healing, thickening agent. It can easily be mixed with fruit juice to make nutrient-dense "Jell-O" cubes, or even marshmallow treats.

Rose water: Used in Rose & Coconut Body Oil (page 220), this delicacy from Middle Eastern cuisine can also be dropped into smoothies and nut milks for a heavenly aromatic twist. It's easy to find in health food stores or Asian markets, and a large bottle is very inexpensive. It's also a wonderful facial cleanser. Keep in the fridge.

Maca powder, spirulina, and bee pollen ($): Though not technically traditional postpartum foods, these three nutritious super food add-ins make smoothies utterly addictive and doubly uplifting. Nutty-tasting maca energizes; emerald-green spirulina feeds and purifies, and golden nuggets of bee pollen—famed as a complete food—deliver fabulous B vitamins along with protein. If you want to treat yourself, add these to your shopping or wish list.

Equipment

An enormous, French chef–style stockpot for broth and a top-of-the-line blender for smoothies and nut milks are wonderful additions to a kitchen, but these advanced accoutrements are not essential. Every recipe in *The First Forty Days* is intended to be achievable without buying extra cookware. Check to see that you have the following kitchen basics and you will be ready to go.

ESSENTIAL KITCHENWARE

- Cooking pots of various sizes, including a large soup/stockpot. If you don't own a large-enough one, bone broth ingredients can be prepared in two smaller pots used simultaneously.

- A thick-bottomed pot, Dutch oven, or a braiser is great for congee and stew.

- A slow cooker, if you have one, can be used for broths, stews, and even congee.

- Steaming basket or colander to steam foods over a pot of boiling water.

- Knives: A chef's knife and a paring knife will do you fine.

- Chopping boards: One for raw meats, one for produce.

- Blender: Any blender that can handle blending softened, soaked nuts will do.

- Cheesecloth or fine-mesh strainer: For filtering your fresh nut milk. Nut milk bags are the pro tool, but not essential. Should you buy one, however, spend a few extra dollars for a bag that doesn't tear and goes the distance.

- A few large mixing bowls for holding ingredients and straining nut milks.

- A funnel: Makes pouring liquids into storage jars infinitely easier.

- Quart- and gallon-size zip-tight plastic bags for freezing portions of soups and stews.

- Storage containers: Tupperware will do, but I prefer glass jars for storing teas/dried goods and glass containers with lids for cooked food/leftovers. Glass is healthier than plastic for storing food items—even compared to BPA-free plastic—as other compounds in plastic are equally dangerous, especially when in contact with hot liquids, and plastic compounds, along with many other environmental toxins, make their way into breast milk. A set of glass storage containers might be the one special kitchen accessory I'd recommend buying—it feels great to know your healthy food is staying that way.

- Muffin tin: A secret weapon for freezing small batches of broths and other foods.

PANTRY RESOURCES

Some of my favorite sources of bulk and specialty items:

- Teas, bulk herbs, spices, and goji berries: mountainroseherbs.com

- Rose water and other hard-to-find ethnic items: shamra.com

- Dried mushrooms: fungusamongus.com, willowharvestorganics.com

- Chinese red dates: teacuppa.com

- Chinese black sweetened vinegar: amazon.com

- Bulk ordered nuts and seeds, including black sesame: shoporganic.com, nuts.com

- Great Lakes gelatin: amazon.com

- Cacao, maca, spirulina, hemp: navitasnaturals.com

- Coconut butter, chia seeds, hemp: nutiva.com

- Bee pollen, royal jelly, raw honey: amazon.com

- Grains, legumes: amazon.com, frontiercoop.com

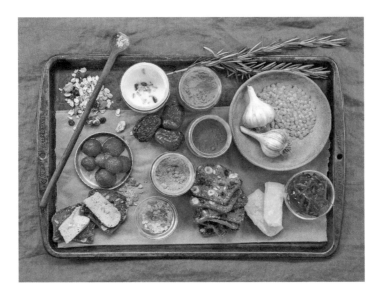

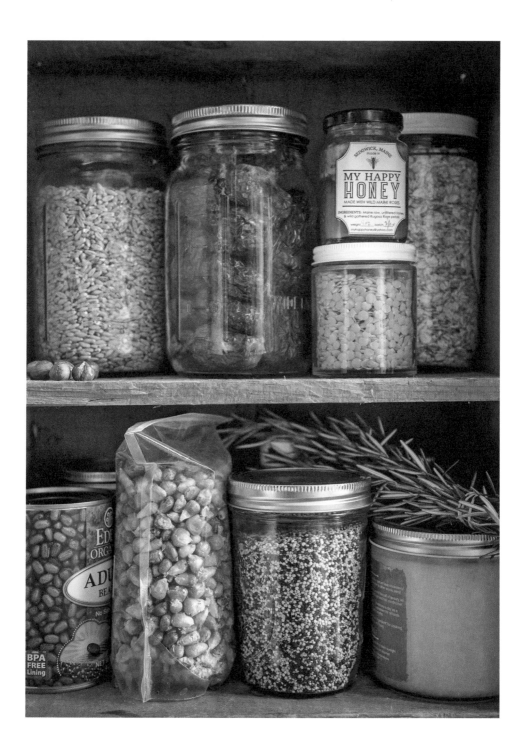

7

the first forty days

recipes

broths

Broth is the first thing I feed a new mother in the days after birth. A sip of this hot and savory liquid will replenish lost energy and bring back some of your power. Time slows down a little. Muscles relax. Heat returns. Everything feels doable again.

I attribute this effect to the incredible nutrients that get infused into this miraculous food—what some call "liquid gold." The oldest records of Chinese healing herald bone broths' power to boost chi and build blood, and restore adrenal function—something that's essential for combating deep-rooted fatigue. Picture how bones support our very being; they are our pillars of strength. The broth that's made by cooking them for hours on end will flood your body with a host of minerals in ultra-absorbable form—essential for every activity in the body—and lots of gelatin, the jelly-like substance in a rich broth that boosts our collagen. It's a boon not just for youth and beauty (think: great hair, skin, and nails) but also helps wounds recover, so if you have stitches of any kind after delivering your baby, definitely drink your broth!

The gelatin is also beloved by your digestive tract, which is why some kind of brothy soup is drunk before every single meal in households led by a Chinese cook. Gelatin helps stoke the fire in your middle burner, the spleen and stomach. Its amino acids help you digest food and even get more protein out of meat, which is a plus if you've splurged on nice grass-fed beef—it'll stretch further. There's more: Bone broth's hydrating power is ideal for breastfeeding. It floods the body with natural electrolytes that are much kinder to the body than bright orange sports drinks. And its lubricating quality counterbalances any vata—airy dryness—in the digestive system, helping to keep your elimination regular as well.

Broth really is the foundation of postpartum eating, and having a stash in your fridge or freezer becomes a lifesaver in the early days with baby. Heat up a saucepan of any variety of broth and add in a medley of protein, vegetables, and noodles. Voilà! The quickest soup in town. Ladle chicken broth into rice to cook a super-warming congee. Or drink it on its own with a splash of Bragg or soy sauce.

The recipes that follow will get you started, but don't take them too literally. Which broth to start with might depend on what ingredients are simplest to source. Most people begin by making chicken broth, then work up to beef—with fish or pork stocks as more adventurous choices. Once you have the feel for it, you can freestyle a bit. Mix and match bones (pork and chicken; beef and lamb) and add any wilting vegetables to extract the last ounce of goodness from the produce you've bought. Broth can be thicker and more protein-filled or thinner and more fluid, depending on the meat and fat on the bones you use. With some experimenting, you'll learn what you like best.

Packaged broth can certainly help you make a roster of recipes, but homemade broth is a world apart. Once you discover how easy it is, you'll be hooked. In terms of cost-to-benefit ratio, broth is a winner, because the several pounds of meat and bones that go into the pot can be reboiled several times to yield quarts of broth that can be used so many ways. And once it's at a simmer, you can walk away for hours. Broth really is your most loyal friend. It's very accepting of your distracted state and doesn't complain if you forget to check in.

BEEF BONE BROTH

THIS IS A WONDERFULLY EARTHY and warming food that requires zero finesse to make. Just handling the ingredients—roughly chopped vegetables, meaty bones that are briefly roasted to boost the flavor, and a dash of vinegar to pull minerals into the liquid—feels primal and earthy. And a mug of broth might just be the perfect food as you shush your little one to sleep; it will keep you going for a couple of hours as its goodness seeps right into *your* bones.

Makes 2 quarts (2 L) or 6–8 servings

4 pounds (1.8 kg) beef bones (short ribs, marrow, neck, joints, whatever you can get)

1 white or yellow onion, halved

2-inch (5-cm) knob of fresh ginger, unpeeled, halved

2 leeks, white parts only, roughly chopped

3 large carrots, unpeeled, sliced into thick rounds

1 tablespoon apple cider vinegar

½ teaspoon whole cloves (optional)

½ teaspoon star anise (optional)

Sea salt and freshly ground black pepper

Preheat the oven to 350°F (175°C).

Place the bones in a large roasting pan (or, if it's ovenproof, in the stockpot that you'll use to cook them on the stove). To save time, add the onions and ginger with the bones so they begin caramelizing as well. (This will give the broth a rich flavor.) Roast for about 30 minutes, or until the bones are brown and crackly and juice has started to collect on the bottom of the pan.

If you used a roasting pan, let the bones cool slightly, then transfer them to a stockpot. Or if you're using the same pot, add 3 quarts (2.8 L) water, or enough to cover the bones with the roasted onion and ginger by about 1 inch (2.5 cm). Add the leeks, carrots, vinegar, and, if using, the cloves and star anise.

Bring to a boil over high heat, skim off any foam that rises to the top, then reduce the heat to low and simmer for 2 to 4 hours, covered, checking every so often to skim off any additional foam. The broth is done when it delivers an appealing earthy flavor.

Remove from the heat, strain, and season with salt and pepper to taste, reserving the bones to make more broth later or immediately add more water and boil the bones again. Drink warm or pour into glass mason jars and keep in the fridge for up to 5 days. (Remember this homemade broth can be used as a component in other recipes— soups, stews, congees—over the next several days.) Or, fill glass mason jars (see page 130), zip-tight plastic bags, or muffin tins (for convenient individual servings) and freeze up to 3 months.

TIP: *To make this broth in a slow cooker, set on medium or low heat and cook for approximately 8 hours. Remove any fat that forms on top.*

OXTAIL BROTH

OXTAIL BONES ARE A BROTH-LOVER'S delight. Robust and fat-rich, oxtail meat falls off the bone into the liquid as it cooks, giving you a delicious gift: slow-cooked beef morsels to snack on. The strips of kombu seaweed infuse satisfying flavor and extra minerals to the liquid. Start cooking oxtail broth in the morning and you can scoop out a few bites of meat midday, letting the broth cook on until evening. There will be more foam on the top of the pot than regular beef broth; simply skim it off.

Makes 2 quarts (2 L) or 6–8 servings

4 pounds (1.8 kg) beef oxtail bones (ask your butcher to help you if you're not familiar)

Sea salt and freshly ground black pepper

1 large white or yellow onion, peeled, quartered

2 strips kombu (helps with digestion and flavor; optional)

1 large daikon, peeled and cut into 1-inch (2.5-cm) slices

3 tablespoons soy sauce, tamari, or Bragg Liquid Aminos

Preheat the oven to 350°F (175°C).

Rinse the oxtail, pat dry, and season with a few pinches of salt and pepper. Place the oxtail and onions in a roasting pan and roast for 30 minutes, or until both the oxtail and the onions are golden brown.

In a large stockpot, bring 3 quarts (2.8 L) water to a boil over medium-high heat. Add the roasted oxtail, roasted onions, and

kombu, if using, leaving the drippings out. Cover the pot, reduce the heat to low, and let simmer for about 2 to 4 hours.

Add the daikon and soy sauce to the broth, then reduce the heat to low and simmer for another hour, covered, or until you see a noticeable reduction in the amount of liquid. (You'll see a ring on the side of the pot when the water level has gone down.)

You'll know the broth is ready when the meat is falling off the bones. You can either eat the broth with the tasty meat in it and suck on the bones, which I love doing, or you can strain out the solids to make a clearer broth.

Store in the fridge for up to 5 days. You can also freeze the broth in zip-tight freezer bags or glass mason jars (see page 130) for up to 3 months.

TIP: *Rich oxtail broth can be customized into a 5-minute noodle bowl. Cook rice noodles, egg noodles, or regular pasta separately—then add to the broth along with flavorings (such as 1 teaspoon Bragg Liquid Aminos or Chinese sweetened black vinegar) and any vegetables you like and eat up!*

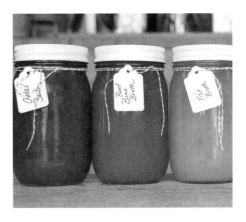

CHICKEN BROTH

NO MATTER WHERE YOU GO in the world, chicken soup fills the new mother's belly. It's nurturing, nourishing, and when you take a sip, it says, "Everything's okay." *Zuo yuezi* prizes chicken for its warming properties, and when combined with also-warming ginger, which boosts circulation and supports your immune system and digestion, chicken soup is an absolute winner for giving your body and soul a cozy glow.

Makes 2 quarts (2 L) or 6–8 servings

2–2½ pounds (1–1.2 kg) whole chicken or parts, organic or free-range preferred

1 medium white or yellow onion, peeled and halved

2-inch (5-cm) knob of fresh ginger, peeled and halved

2 whole garlic cloves, peeled

2 whole green onion stalks

2 medium carrots, not peeled, sliced into medium rounds

Sea salt and freshly ground pepper

Rinse the chicken under cold running water, then place the chicken carcass or pieces in a large pot with 3 quarts (2.8 L) cold water, enough to cover the chicken by at least 1 inch (2.5 cm). Bring to a boil over medium-high heat, reduce to a low simmer, and simmer for about 30 minutes. Skim off any scum as it rises to the top.

Add the onion, ginger, garlic, green onions, and carrots and cook over medium heat, then let the broth cook for another 3 hours on low heat, uncovered. Season to taste with salt and pepper. The meat will slowly separate and fall off the bones. Strain, or if you want to portion out some broth with meat and vegetables to eat as a chunky soup, you can do that now.

Store leftovers in the fridge for up to 5 days, or freeze in zip-tight plastic bags or glass mason jars (see below) for up to 3 months.

TIP: *If chicken feet are available from your butcher, add several to the pot. It'll boost the broth further, giving you a richer liquid and heartier mouthfeel. When the broth cools in the fridge, it may congeal into jelly, due to the high gelatin content. Scoop a few spoonfuls of this into almost anything you're making (grains, soups, vegetables) to add moisture, while enhancing taste and nutrition. It will clarify into liquid when heated.*

HOW TO FREEZE BROTH

To freeze broth in glass mason jars: Pour the cooled broth into a clean jar, leaving 2 inches (5 cm) headspace at the top. Screw the lids on loosely and place them in the freezer with a little space between each jar (this will help prevent cracked jars). Once the broth is frozen, you can tighten the lids. Freeze for up to 3 months. To defrost, place a jar or two in the fridge the night before. Heat the contents in a pot on the stovetop as needed.

PORK & DAIKON BROTH

TWO HUMBLE INGREDIENTS—PORK
BONES and daikon radish, which
helps to break down meat protein—
combined with a splurge ingredient,
fresh or dried shiitakes, will deliver
a broth that is as delicious as it is
digestible. Adding the pork shoulder
will infuse the broth with extra flavor
while giving you a batch of super-tasty
shredded pork to store separately in
the fridge. You can stir it back into
the broth to make a hearty soup, or
use it in a congee recipe (pages 155-
156, Seaweed Soup (page 147), or a
Mother's Bowl (page 167).

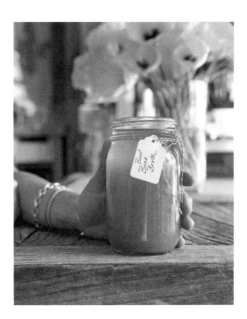

Makes 2 quarts (2 L) or 6–8 servings

4 pounds (1.8 kg) pork bones plus 1 pound
  (455 g) pork butt, if available, halved

1 large white or yellow onion, peeled and
  halved

Sea salt and freshly ground black pepper

2 strips kombu (helps with digestion and
  flavor)

2 cups (85 g) fresh shiitake mushrooms,
  or 1 cup (35 g) dried

1 pound (455 g) bacon (optional)

4 whole green onion stalks, washed

1 cup (115 g) thinly sliced daikon rounds

2 large carrots, peeled and roughly chopped

Preheat the oven to 400°F (205°C).

Place the pork bones, pork butt, and
onions in a roasting pan, season with a few
pinches of salt and pepper and roast for
30 minutes, or until the bones and butt are

golden brown and juices begin to form at the
bottom of the pan.

In a large stockpot, add 3 quarts (2.8 L)
cold water and the kombu and let it come to
a boil. Reduce the heat to medium, then add
the shiitake mushrooms and bacon, if using.

Remove the bones, butt, and onion from
the oven and transfer to the stockpot with
the broth. Add the green onions, daikon, and
carrots. Let it all simmer over medium heat for
30 minutes, uncovered, then reduce to low
heat for 3 hours. Skim off any foam as it rises
to the top.

Season to taste with more salt and
pepper. Strain, or if you want to portion out
some of the broth with meat and vegetables
to eat as a chunky soup, you can do that now.

Store leftovers in the fridge for up to 5
days, or freeze in airtight plastic bags or glass
mason jars (see page 130) for up to 3 months.

FISH BROTH

LIGHT AND AROMATIC, FISH BROTH is a wonderfully adaptable kitchen classic that is often overlooked in the West. In Asia, it's a base for soups, stews, and ramen bowls because it accommodates all kinds of flavorings quite easily. Experiment with this broth: Add your favorite spices to change its personality—try allspice for a Vietnamese twist—or omit the tomatoes to make a clear, multi-purpose broth.

If it's your first time buying a whole fish with the head on, don't be intimidated. It's an economical choice (and rewarding, as the head has tons of flavor and nutrients) and the fishmonger will typically wash and prep it for you. Small bones may be left inside; they will soften when cooked and contain extra nutrition—just pick them out before eating or chew well!

Makes 2 quarts (2 L) or 6–8 servings

1 medium white or yellow onion, peeled and halved

1 clove garlic, peeled and roughly chopped

1-inch (2.5-cm) knob of fresh ginger, unpeeled, halved

4 green onions, roots trimmed

2 medium tomatoes, unpeeled, halved

2 pounds (910 g) whole fish with heads and tails (see Tip, next column)

1 tablespoon unsweetened black vinegar

1 cup fresh (165 g) or frozen (245 g) pineapple (optional for a sweetener)

Sea salt and pepper

Place the onion, garlic, ginger, green onions, and tomatoes in a medium pot. Add 3 quarts (2.8 L) water, or enough to cover everything by at least 1 inch (2.5 cm). Bring to a boil, then reduce the heat and simmer, covered, for 30 minutes.

Add the fish, vinegar, and pineapple, if using, raise the heat, and bring it to a gentle boil, skimming off any foam as it rises. Reduce the heat to a simmer and cook gently for 45 minutes, uncovered.

When the liquid becomes cloudy, remove from heat and strain the remnants through a cheesecloth or metal strainer, separating the broth into a clean jar or bowl and discarding the solids. Season to taste with salt and pepper.

This broth is best enjoyed very fresh, so set aside what you can use in a day and freeze the rest in zip-tight plastic bags or glass mason jars (see page 130) for up to 3 months.

TIP: *You can also use meaty white or dark fish such as cod, sea bass, or halibut, but whole fish with the bones and head are best. They add the most nutrition to the broth, plus it's cheaper to buy fish that way.*

THE ART OF SITTING STILL

Once the adrenaline from birth has faded and the buzz surrounding baby's arrival has quieted, you may find yourself facing an unforeseen, and often undiscussed, challenge of brand-new parenthood: boredom. The baby books usually skip this topic—who wants to read a chapter called "The Monotony of Motherhood"?—but it's a key part of these first weeks with baby. You're on what seems like an endless loop of nurse-burp-rock-repeat, and the sameness may initially be quite challenging, tedious, even.

In fact, when your partner goes back to work and the stream of visitors slows to a trickle, you may find that your role as primary caretaker for a helpless, miniature human being requires a level of stamina that surpasses bouncing your wailing wee one for more than an hour on a rubbery exercise ball or making it through five days with no more than two consecutive hours of sleep. As the only food source for your baby and his numero-uno path to comfort and security, your job is endless. But—surprise!—your job description neglected to mention that you will spend much of that time sitting. Whether you're sitting in bed propped up by pillows, sitting on the couch, or sitting in a comfy chair, you will dedicate the bulk of your time during the first forty days with your new baby to feeding him (this goes for bottle-fed babies, too)—which is most easily accomplished in a seated position. If this is your first baby, especially, you may find all this sitting still disconcerting. This is another example of the paradox of the Gateway. These early weeks with baby are inherently stimulating as you activate your mind and intuition in an effort to shape his various cries and movements into some type of decipherable baby language. And they're emotionally fulfilling as you ride the waves of oxytocin released when you nurse your babe and when you cuddle or kiss her. Yet your time with baby can feel like a marathon of near-nothingness.

As you settle in for yet another nursing session, sitting in the same chair facing the same tree framed by the same window, you may find yourself wondering how the most special time of your life can also be so boring. Though he's growing and changing fast, your baby is not the most engaging company. You may feel lonely or antsy or blue.

This is good news! These feelings are signs that you are at an exciting crossroads. You can choose to drown out the simplicity of this time with TV, your smart phone—which should also be kept far away from baby's head to prevent exposure to dangerous EMFs—or other distractions, or you can use it as an opportunity to be present and give your full attention to the here and now—without judging it or attaching any kind of story to it. Begin to notice, really notice, as much as you can about each moment with baby in your arms. It may seem like not much is happening—you're just sitting in a chair nursing your baby—but every moment contains an entire world of experience. Notice the satisfied little grunts baby makes while nursing. Notice the sound of the wind ruffling the leaves of the tree outside your window. Notice the dull ache in your lower back. Notice the sweetness you feel in your heart when baby plays with your hair or grasps onto your finger. These individual moments add up to a richer experience than you may have realized. Suddenly what seemed like a whole lot of nothing is actually quite something.

SHIITAKE IMMUNE-BOOST BROTH

WITH A NEWBORN NEEDING ALL your attention and care, it's more important than ever to protect yourself from colds and keep your immune system strong. This meat-free broth benefits from the immune-boosting power of mushrooms—long revered in Chinese medicine as a powerful medicinal food. Rich in B vitamins and minerals, they seduce the senses with a smoky flavor. Shiitake broth can go head to head with beef broth in taste. With its satisfying, savory tang, it's like the Portobello burger to a carnivore's hamburger.

Makes 2 quarts (2 L) or 6–8 servings

1 white or yellow onion, peeled and roughly chopped

2 leeks, green parts discarded, white part roughly chopped into coin shapes

2 tablespoons olive oil or a cooking oil like avocado or coconut oil or grass-fed butter

Sea salt

2 cups (85 g) fresh shiitake mushrooms, or 1 cup (35 g) dried

½ cup (20 g) dried reishi mushrooms (optional)

1 cup (60 g) cremini or white button mushrooms

2 strips kombu (helps with digestion and flavor)

2 medium carrots, peeled and roughly chopped

4 medium tomatoes, halved, with seeds is fine

3 whole cloves garlic, peeled

1-inch (2.5-cm) knob of fresh turmeric, unpeeled, halved

2 cups (140 g) roughly chopped green cabbage

1 loosely packed cup (50 g) roughly chopped parsley

2 tablespoons lemon zest

In a medium pot over medium heat, brown the onions and leeks in the oil with a pinch of sea salt to help the browning.

Quickly rinse the shiitake, reishi (if using), and cremini mushrooms and kombu under running water. Add all the mushrooms, kombu, carrots, tomatoes, garlic, and turmeric to the pot, along with 3 quarts (2.8 L) water, or enough water to cover the veggies by at least 1 inch (2.5 cm). Cook for 1 hour over medium-low heat, covered. During the last 20 minutes, add the cabbage, parsley, and lemon zest.

Season the broth to taste with salt. Remove from heat and strain.

Store in the fridge for up to 5 days, or freeze in zip-tight plastic bags or glass mason jars (see page 130) for up to 3 months.

TIP: *Chilled cabbage leaves can provide relief for hard or sore breasts. Store in refrigerator, pull off individual leaves, and place directly on breasts for ten minutes. Repeat as necessary. Continue to nurse or pump, drink lots of water, and, most essential: get more sleep, as sleep deprivation is almost always the number-one cause. A clogged milk duct may feel hard in one spot. Massage gently with a warm compress or under the shower, and try homeopathic remedies Phytolacca 30c (for hardness) and Belladonna 30c (if fever occurs). If you suspect mastitis infection be sure to consult your health-care provider.*

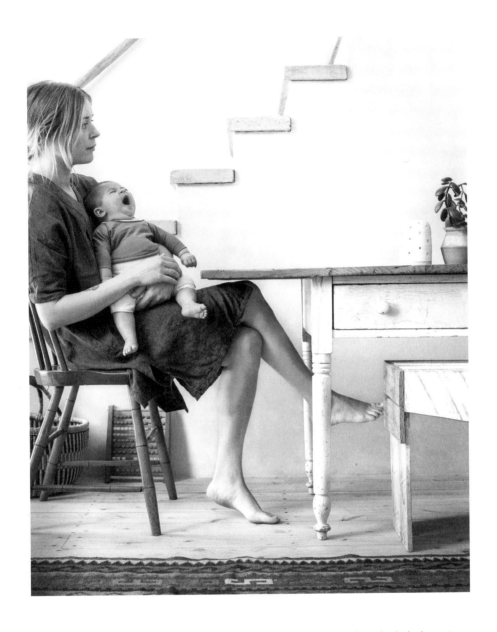

All the baby really has are its eyes and ears—its senses—and its inhale and exhale. Its entire experience is made up of the present moment. So how beautiful to be able to connect with yourself in that very same way and in doing so, connect fully with what your baby is experiencing.

—JENNA HUMPHREYS, LM, CPM, REGISTERED MIDWIFE, DOULA, AND PLACENTA ENCAPSULATIONIST, SANTA BARBARA, CA

soups & stews

Soup is the food that makes a new mother feel loved. It's the simplest nourishment, yet it has such an impact. Delivering a container of homemade soup for a woman who's alone with her newborn is like putting TLC into edible form. It says that you see what she's just gone through, and you see what she needs right now. And that dose of TLC can be exchanged without a word—just warm up the soup and serve with a smile.

If you are a new mom, chances are you will start to make many of your own meals sometime into the postpartum process. Soup's great for that as well. It's the most basic kind of cooking, just one step more involved than making broth. Gather your ingredients, throw them in the pot with liquid, light the flame, and let the heat bring out the flavors. You don't need a lot of fancy flourishes to make it taste good. This isn't the haute cuisine school of soup making. A few quality ingredients, and enough time, will provide warming, nourishing sustenance. As you get familiar with making soup, you can customize what goes into it depending on what's on hand or what you feel your body needs—more meat one day, more greens the next. The matriarchs of kitchens past used a free hand, tossing in goji berries if mom's eyes looked dull or seaweed if she seemed wan. Get to know the things that feel good for your body and spirit as you eat, then channel a little of this matriarchal confidence as you cook.

The soups in this section run the gamut: from clear and light to mushy and soft, to stews with a little more heft that feed an especially hungry stomach and satisfy everyone in the family. Whether you're making these yourself or letting a loved one do the work, these recipes are straightforward and flexible, and shouldn't be an effort.

As you collect your ingredients, or as your sister chops and your best friend stirs, take a moment and notice if you feel the lineage of women who have done exactly this, in their kitchens, throughout time. Know that you are part of history's rich story of mothering, with all its joys and challenges. You are not alone.

QUINOA, LENTILS & GREENS SOUP

SOME TRADITIONAL POSTPARTUM SOUPS ARE elaborate concoctions requiring many steps and rare ingredients. This soup is the opposite: a super-simple meal made from basic pantry ingredients that's impossible to get wrong. The spices and flavorings can be intensified as you like. Adding nutritional yeast will give you a boost of B vitamins plus the addictive savory taste known as "umami."

Serves 8

¾ cup (85 g) peeled and roughly chopped white or yellow onion

3 tablespoons olive oil or coconut oil

Sea salt

2 quarts (2 L) homemade broth (see pages 128-132) or use store-bought

2 tablespoons ground cumin

4 medium carrots, peeled, quartered, and cut into small cubes

2 cups (400 g) green lentils

1½ cups (255 g) quinoa

3 cups (195 g) roughly chopped curly kale (stems included)

1 tablespoon soy sauce, tamari, or Bragg Liquid Aminos

3 tablespoons nutritional yeast (optional)

In a medium pot over medium heat, sauté the onions in the oil with a pinch of salt until they brown on the edges and are tender.

Add the broth, cumin, carrots, and lentils, bring to a boil over high heat, then reduce the heat to medium-low and cook, stirring occasionally, 30 to 40 minutes, or until the carrots and lentils have begun to soften. Add the quinoa and kale, reduce the heat to a simmer, and cook for another 15 minutes, covered, until the quinoa is cooked and the kale is tender.

Remove from heat, season with the soy sauce and the nutritional yeast, if using, and stir in a pinch of salt, or season to taste.

Serve warm. Store leftovers in a glass storage container in the fridge for 3 to 4 days. This soup also freezes well for up to 3 months, portioned into zip-tight plastic bags or glass mason jars (see page 130).

CHICKEN, RED DATES & GINGER SOUP

THIS TWIST ON A CLASSIC "first food" for mom may sound strange. Dried fruit in chicken soup, you ask? But go with it: Chinese red dates—also known as jujubes, available at Chinese markets or online—plus ruby-colored goji berries is a time-tested combo used to boost circulation and enhance inner warmth. Your eyes will delight at the look of these little gems in your soup bowl. Your taste buds will love the subtle touch of sweetness against the savory chicken. I recommend making every effort to use Chinese red dates, which bestow amazing postpartum health benefits, as they are not difficult to find online or in local Asian markets. Medjool dates are okay in a pinch but they do not have the same medicinal effects.

Serves 6–8

2–2½ pounds (1–1.2 kg) whole chicken or parts, organic or free-range preferred

½ of a white or yellow onion, peeled

2-inch (5-cm) knob of fresh ginger, unpeeled, halved

3 medium carrots, peeled and thinly sliced

5 Chinese red dates (see "Pantry Resources," page 124)

3 tablespoons dried goji berries (see "Pantry Resources," page 124)

Sea salt

Rinse the chicken under cold water, place in a medium stockpot, and add enough cold water to just cover the chicken. Bring to a boil over medium-high heat, uncovered.

Once boiling, add the onion and ginger to the pot. Reduce heat to medium and cook for 40 minutes, covered. Every so often, remove the lid to skim any foam off the top and discard.

Remove from heat, and with the help of tongs, remove the chicken and set it aside to cool. When cool enough to handle, remove the cooked meat from the carcass and shred it. Return the rest of the carcass to the pot. Add 1–2 cups of the shredded meat (reserving the rest for another use), along with the carrots and red dates, and simmer over low heat, uncovered, for 1 hour. Set a timer to go off in the last 15 minutes, and stir in the goji berries. Season with a pinch or two of salt, or more, to taste.

Drink this soup throughout the day, keep in the fridge for up to 5 days, or freeze in zip-tight plastic bags or glass mason jars (see page 130) for up to 3 months.

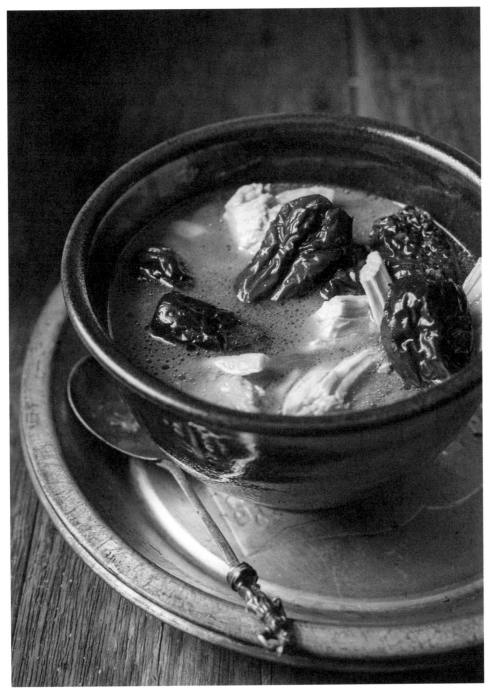

Chicken, Red Dates & Ginger Soup

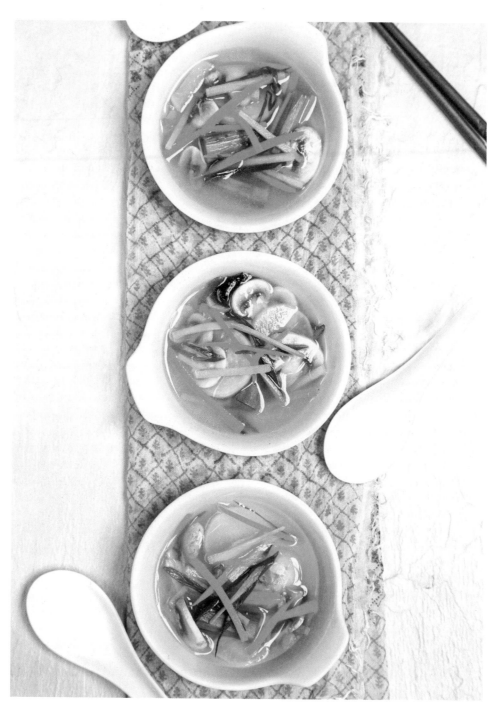

Miso & Burdock Soup

MISO & BURDOCK SOUP

DRINKING THIS SOUP WHEN COCOONED in your little nest will feel like getting a hug from Mother Nature. Combine burdock root, mushrooms, seaweed, and salty miso paste in a pot, and you get a fortifying balance of land and sea. Fresh burdock root is famed for its purifying and immune-boosting effects and can be found at health food stores and Asian markets.

Serves 6

1-inch (2.5-cm) knob of fresh ginger, peeled and sliced into matchsticks

1 cup (60 g) matchsticks of fresh unpeeled burdock (if fresh is not available, you can use ½ cup (about 80 g) dried burdock)

1 cup (115 g) cubes of unpeeled daikon

1 medium carrot, peeled and cut into cubes

2 whole green onions, white ends cut off and discarded

1 cup (70 g) sliced white or (60 g) cremini mushrooms

1 strip of kombu (helps with digestion and flavor)

2 tablespoons sesame oil

2 teaspoons organic miso of choice

In a medium stockpot, bring 7 cups (1.7 L) water to a rolling boil. Add the ginger, burdock, daikon, carrots, green onions, mushrooms, kombu, and sesame oil, reduce heat to low, and simmer, covered, for 40 minutes. Remove from heat.

Spoon out some of the hot broth into a small bowl, stir in the miso paste, and let it dissolve.

When the rest of the broth has cooled a bit and the steam has subsided, after about 5 minutes, stir the miso broth back into the pot.

This is a great soup to drink throughout the day as needed. Pour the desired amount of soup into a smaller pot and reheat it on the lowest setting, without letting it come to a boil (that will destroy the enzymes in the miso). Soup can be stored in the fridge up to 5 days.

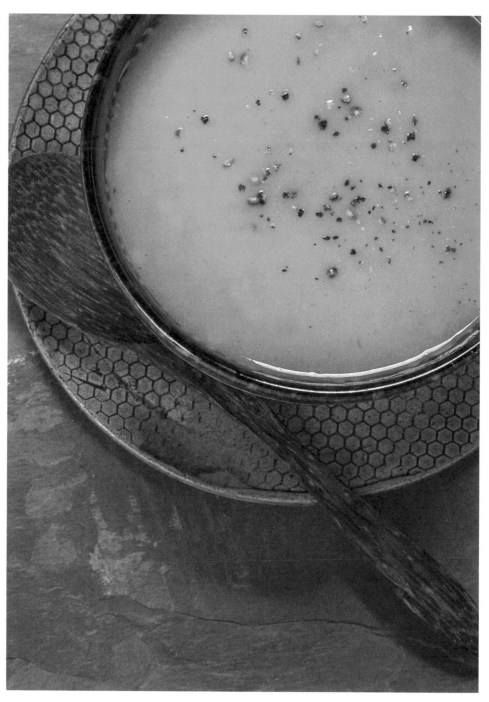

Creamy Kabocha & Red Lentil Soup

CREAMY KABOCHA & RED LENTIL SOUP

ORANGE IS A COLOR OF celebration, ritual, and happiness—a shade that instantly lifts the spirits. This pureed soup is so easy to make from ingredients stocked in your pantry, and it's a great one to ask a visitor to whip up for you. The slightly sweet taste and grounding properties of kabocha squash are especially comforting on days when you might feel teary or blue, and a generous amount of lubricating oil helps to remedy inner dryness and wind, soothing the nerves further. Combine this soup with the Oxtail Stew (page 149) for a wonderfully rich and satisfying concoction.

Serves 8

3 tablespoons sesame oil or coconut oil

½ of a white or yellow onion, peeled and roughly chopped

½ of a shallot, roughly chopped

1 medium kabocha squash, peeled and cut into small cubes (6 cups/690 g), or substitute acorn or butternut squash

1 teaspoon ground cumin

1 tablespoon curry powder

2 quarts (2 L) vegetable broth (Shiitake Immune-Boost Broth, page 134, or store-bought)

2 cups (380 g) red lentils

2 teaspoons soy sauce, tamari, or Bragg Liquid Aminos, or to taste

2 tablespoons nutritional yeast (optional)

Warm the oil in a large pot over medium heat. Add the onion and shallot and lightly brown them, stirring with a wooden spoon, about 5 minutes. Add the squash, cumin, and curry powder and lightly sauté with the onions, about 5 minutes more.

Reduce heat to medium-low, add the broth, and bring to a boil. Cover the pot, reduce heat to low, and cook for 40 minutes. Add the lentils and continue to cook for another 10 to 15 minutes, until the lentils and squash are tender.

Let the soup cool slightly, then transfer it to a blender in batches and puree until creamy, if you like, or stop when some of the squash is still chunky. (Or use a hand blender to blend the soup in the pot.) Season with the soy sauce and nutritional yeast, if using, to taste.

Drink throughout the day. Store leftovers in the fridge for up to 5 days, or freeze in zip-tight plastic bags or glass mason jars (see page 130) for up to 3 months.

SEASONAL GREENS SOUP

IT'S HARD FOR ANYONE TO get their daily serving of fortifying greens, let alone a new mom! And since you're avoiding cold raw salads (per the Five Insights of the First Forty Days; see number 2, warmth, page 33), it may seem doubly tough to get your greens on—but there are definitely quick and warming options available. This soup helps to address that conundrum. By simmering and liquefying lots of leaves at once, you can consume a gardenful of greens in one brightly colored and very easily digestible bowl. Quinoa boosts the soup by adding texture, protein, and a pop of contrasting color. Seasonal Greens Soup has an essential role in the new mom's repertoire.

Serves 6—8

3 leeks, white parts only, cut crosswise into thin slices

½ cup (55 g) peeled and roughly chopped white or yellow onion

3 medium parsnips, peeled and roughly chopped

3 tablespoons olive oil or coconut oil

2 quarts (2 L) vegetable broth (Shiitake Immune-Boost Broth, page 134, or store-bought)

½ teaspoon sea salt

1 cup (170 g) quinoa

3 loosely packed cups (90 g) fresh organic spinach

1 loosely packed cup (30 g) chopped chard

2 tablespoons soy sauce, tamari, or Bragg Liquid Aminos, or to taste

2 tablespoons nutritional yeast (optional)

In a large pot over medium-high heat, sauté the leeks, onions, and parsnips in the oil until lightly browned. Add the broth, reduce the heat to medium, cover, and let it simmer for about 30 minutes, or until the parsnips are soft.

Meanwhile, in a small pot, bring 2 cups (480 ml) water and the salt to a gentle boil. Add the quinoa, reduce the heat, and simmer, covered, for 15 minutes, or until the quinoa is fluffy and tender and has unfurled (opened) slightly.

When the soup has finished cooking, remove it from the heat to cool down a bit. Working in batches, transfer the warm soup to a blender, along with the fresh spinach and chard, and blend until everything is incorporated into a vibrant green puree (or use a hand blender).

Return the puree to the pot, stir in the quinoa, and season with the soy sauce and the nutritional yeast, if using.

Warm up the soup over low heat before serving. Store leftovers in the fridge for up to 5 days, or freeze in zip-tight plastic bags or glass mason jars (see page 130) for up to 3 months.

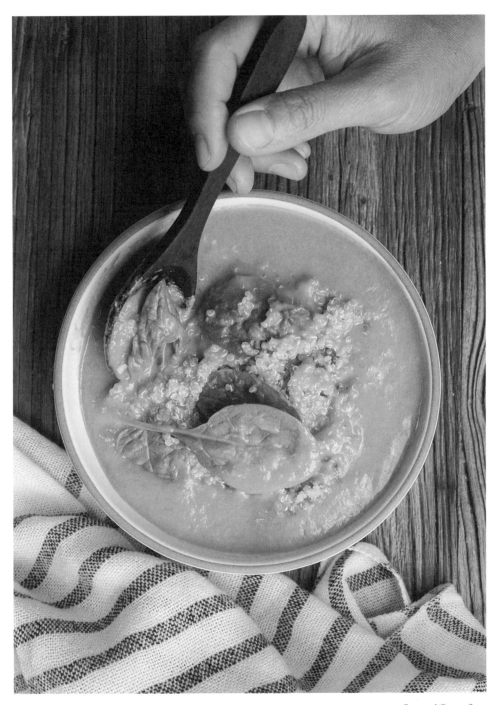

Seasonal Greens Soup

POSTPARTUM EGG-DROP SOUP WITH LIVER & GREENS

THIS LIGHT AND REPLENISHING SOUP is a balance of three superb foods and an effortless way to eat a few bites of healing chicken liver. A cracked-in egg cooks quickly in feathery strands, swirling and tangling into the greens. The small chunks of liver add an earthy, grounding flavor and have a soft and appealing texture; it is not at all hard to chew, like some meat can be. Like all egg-drop soups, this version is best eaten fresh. Make sure to source local and organic organ meat.

Serves 3–4

2 tablespoons minced shallots

3 tablespoons sesame oil

Sea salt

1 clove garlic, minced

2 green onions, root ends trimmed off

4 cups (960 ml) water or broth

1 handful of rice noodles or your favorite
    pasta (optional)

2 large pasture-raised eggs

6 organic chicken livers, rinsed and cut into
    2-inch (5-cm) slices

1 tablespoon ground paprika (or chili powder
    if you want some heat)

3 loosely packed cups (about 105 g) fresh
    greens (watercress, chard, baby kale, or
    organic spinach, whatever you have on
    hand)

1 tablespoon soy sauce, tamari, or Bragg
    Liquid Aminos

In a small pot over medium-low heat, sauté the shallots in the oil with a pinch of salt until the shallots turn soft. Add the garlic, green onions, and water or broth, raise the heat to medium high, and cook at a rolling boil for 5 minutes, uncovered.

Meanwhile, if using noodles, cook them separately in a small pot per instructions on the package. Drain the noodles and divide them among individual soup bowls and set aside.

Reduce heat to low. Whisk the eggs in a small bowl, and then gently pour them into the soup. With a fork or whisk, swirl them in a clockwise direction so they cook while swirling, about 5 minutes more, uncovered.

Add the chicken livers to the pot and cook for another 7 to 10 minutes, covered, until the liver is brown and tender when pierced with a fork. Check it at 5 minutes, as overcooked liver won't taste as good. (Depending on the size of the slices, it may cook faster than expected.)

Add the paprika, greens, and the soy sauce, plus more salt if desired, turn off the heat, and let sit for 5 minutes, covered, so the greens cook in the steam. Pour soup over the noodles, if using, and serve hot.

TIP: *You can "drop" an egg into any light soup. Crack and whisk it in a small bowl, then swirl the egg into the hot liquid with a fork or whisk. It's an instant way to add an extra hit of protein and saturated fat to broth- or water-based soups— and it's really fun as well!*

SEAWEED SOUP

IN KOREA, IT'S TRADITIONAL TO feed a mother *miyeokguk*, or seaweed soup, up to three times a day after she gives birth, because seaweed helps to promote lactation, support the hormones, and calm the nervous system. It makes sense that eating sea vegetables would help in an emotionally charged time. On an energetic level, seaweed reminds us that everything is tidal and constantly changing. It invites us to surrender to the waves and let feelings wash over us. Use any kind of seaweed you like and sip the soup straight up, or doctor it up with beef, rice, and eggs to make a more substantial bowl.

Serves 6–8

½ of a white or yellow onion, peeled and finely chopped

2 tablespoons sesame oil

4 ounces (115 g) beef sirloin, cubed (omit for a vegetarian version), or add 1 cup dried anchovies

1 clove garlic, finely chopped

1 teaspoon sea salt

2 quarts (2 L) water or broth of your choice

2 cups (30 g) dried seaweed (dulse, wakame, hijiki, arame, or kelp), rinsed to remove any residual bits of rocks or shells

6 shiitake mushrooms, dried or fresh

1 tablespoon soy sauce, tamari, or Bragg Liquid Aminos, or to taste

For a heartier stew, add one or all of the following:

1 pound (455 g) organic beef or pork stew meat

½ cup (about 120 g) leftover cooked grains (such as millet or rice)

2 large pasture-raised eggs

In a medium pot over medium heat, sauté the onions in the oil until lightly browned. Add the beef sirloin, garlic, and salt. Stir and cook the meat until it turns a light brown.

Add the water or broth, seaweed, and mushrooms, along with the stew meat and/ or leftover rice, if you want a heartier stew. Reduce the heat to low and let everything simmer, covered, for 40 minutes. If you're adding the eggs, beat them in a small bowl and, about 5 minutes before the soup is done, pour them into the soup, swirling them with a fork or whisking in a clockwise direction as they cook.

Eat warm. Store leftovers in the fridge for up to 3 days, or freeze in zip-tight plastic bags or glass mason jars (see page 130) for up to 3 months.

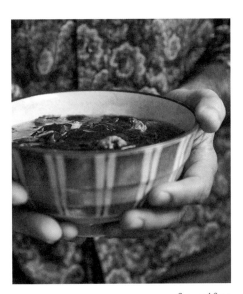

Seaweed Soup

HEARTY SAUSAGE STEW

WHEN THE BELLY IS RUMBLING, a bowl of rustic folk food is in order. This simple-to-make sausage stew is a winner for a hungry mom and her equally hungry helper in the home. It's hearty in feel and flavor and will take whatever sausage you want to use; try a spicier sausage like chorizo—or harissa-spiced lamb merguez if you can find it—to add more flavor and a warming kick. This stew has the greens mixed in, so everything you need is in one big bowl. Serve over a generous heap of couscous or millet and let the grains soak up the sauce.

Serves 6–8

¼ cup (60 ml) cooking oil (coconut, avocado, or animal fat like lard or butter)

Sea salt

½ of a white or yellow onion, roughly chopped

6 medium fresh tomatoes, quartered, with seeds left in (if you don't have fresh, you can use one 15-ounce/430-g can of whole organic tomatoes and their juices)

6 small red potatoes, unpeeled, cut into cubes (about 4 cups/560 g)

2 cups (150 g) quartered mushrooms

2 quarts (2 L) broth of choice (see homemade options, pages 128-132, or use store-bought)

3–5 tablespoons (50–85 g) tomato paste

4 cloves garlic, roughly chopped

3 slices Parmesan cheese rind (adds depth of flavor, optional)

4 sausages (1 pound/455 g) cut into 2-inch (5-cm) sections

1 cup (about 200 g) Israeli couscous or millet

3 large handfuls Swiss chard or 1 bunch spinach, roughly chopped (6–8 cups/180–240 g)

Freshly ground black pepper

In a large pot, over medium-low heat, warm the oil with a pinch of salt. When it's hot, add the onions and cook for 5 minutes, or until they start to brown lightly. Add the tomatoes and potatoes, stirring occasionally to keep the potatoes from sticking to the bottom of the pot. After about 3 minutes, add the mushrooms and cook, stirring occasionally, for 10 minutes.

Add the broth, tomato paste, garlic, and the Parmesan rind, if using, cover the pot, and cook for 1½ hours, on low heat. During the last 15 to 20 minutes, add the sausage along with the couscous (15 minutes) or millet (20 minutes), if using, and cook, covered, then add the chard and cook until it has wilted. Remove from heat and season with salt and pepper to taste.

Serve hot. Store leftovers in the fridge for up to 5 days, or freeze in zip-tight plastic bags or glass mason jars (see page 130) for up to 3 months.

OXTAIL STEW

I LOVE TO COME INTO a mother's kitchen and prepare buttery and succulent oxtail stew as baby naps nearby. It is a slow-cooking dish that takes time and patience—but not much skill or effort. A classic of Jamaican cooking, oxtail stew should really be made with a Bob Marley soundtrack reminding you that "every little thing gonna be alright." This humble meat is a prime example of what used to be called "peasant food"—the least chic and cheapest cut of meat available—but now it's trendy again, so you may have to tussle for it at the butcher case. Ask a savvy friend to procure the meat and make the stew as a gift to your partner and you. Jamaicans serve it with lima beans and rice, but it'll be delicious over clouds of mashed potatoes, polenta (cooked according to package directions), or with rice (you choose the type) and goat cheese.

Serves 6–8

3 tablespoons (45 ml) olive oil, plus more if needed

1 cup (110 g) roughly chopped white or yellow onion

6 loosely packed cups (450 g) sliced or quartered mushrooms

Sea salt and freshly ground pepper

4 pounds (1.8 kg) bone-in oxtails, any and all sizes

2 quarts (2 L) homemade (see page 129) or store-bought broth

2 tablespoons soy sauce, tamari, or Bragg Liquid Aminos

4 small to medium ripe tomatoes, quartered, with seeds left in

2 large carrots, unpeeled, cut into thick slices

1 clove garlic, minced

4 pinches of fresh thyme or 2 pinches of dried thyme (optional)

For the roux (optional):

6 tablespoons (85 g) salted grass-fed butter, at room temperature

6 tablespoons (45 g) all-purpose flour

In a large pot, heat the oil over medium heat. Brown the onions and mushrooms until they turn a golden brown. Turn off the heat and transfer the mushrooms and onions to a small bowl and set aside. Season the oxtail bones with sea salt and pepper and place into the pot until the edges brown slightly, about 10 minutes. Add the tomatoes, carrots, garlic, and thyme, if using, along with the sauteed mushrooms and onions. Let simmer for another 2 hours over low heat, covered. If the meat has not fallen off the bones yet but the liquid has decreased, add more broth or water and continue cooking until it does. Turn off the heat, then season the stew with salt and pepper to taste.

If you would like a thicker stew, make a butter and flour roux: In a small pot, heat the butter over medium-high heat. Whisk in the flour and mix until it starts to bubble. Reduce heat to low and turn the whisking into a gentle stir. Fold the roux into the oxtail stew.

RECIPE CONTINUED ON PAGE 150

RECIPE CONTINUED FROM PAGE 149

Although it's ready to eat hot, the leftovers are the best. Store in the fridge for up to 5 days, or freeze in 2-cup (455-g) portions in zip-tight plastic bags or glass mason jars for up to 3 months.

TIP: *Oxtail will do very well in a slow cooker. Cook on low heat for 4–6 hours, adding more liquid, as needed, until the meat falls off the bones. Scoop off the fat on top after cooking, or after it cools and congeals in the fridge.*

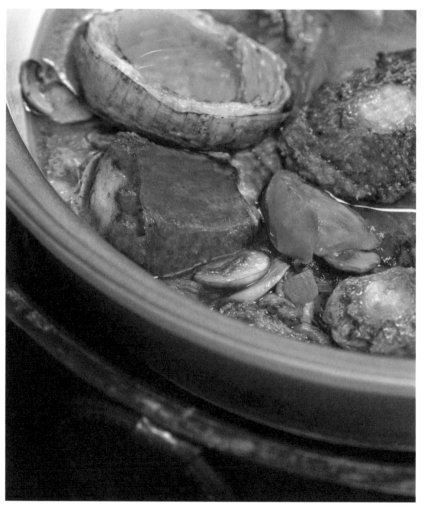

Oxtail Stew

C-RECOVERY VEGETABLE STEW

THE BEAUTY OF THIS VEGETABLE stew is the creative freedom it offers. You can add whatever fresh produce you have to this basic recipe because it will lovingly embrace almost any combination of vegetables. You can eat it many times in a row without tiring of it, and throw in proteins like cooked chicken or sausage if your body desires them. And it's a great meal to ask visiting friends or your partner to help with. Anyone can chop carrots or wash and slice leeks under your gentle guidance, as you sway side to side with baby. I particularly love it for moms who've given birth by cesarean section, because it is so gentle on the digestion and contains some nurturing and lubricating saturated fats. If you are scheduled for a C-section, make this soup ahead of time and freeze it.

Serves 6–8

3 tablespoons ghee or grass-fed butter

1 white or yellow onion, roughly chopped

2 leeks, white parts only, thinly sliced

Sea salt

4 medium carrots, peeled and cut into cubes

3 medium russet potatoes, peeled and cut into cubes

4 medium tomatoes, cut into cubes, keeping as much juice as possible to add to stew

2 cups (140 g) loosely packed mushrooms, quartered

1 tablespoon ground cumin

2 cinnamon sticks

1 cup (120 g) raw cashews

1 tablespoon coriander seeds

1 teaspoon ground turmeric

1 thin slice of ginger (about the length of your pinkie finger)

1 dried bay leaf

6 cups (1.4 L) vegetable broth or water

1½ cups (300 g) millet

1 cup (240 ml) canned coconut milk

1 large handful of green beans

Juice of half a lemon

Heat the ghee or butter in a medium pot over medium-high heat. When it's hot, add the onions and leeks with a pinch of salt, stirring frequently, until the vegetables are golden brown and are tender, about 10 minutes.

Add the carrots, potatoes, tomatoes and their juices, mushrooms, cumin, cinnamon sticks, cashews, coriander seeds, turmeric, ginger, and bay leaf to the pot, along with the broth. Bring to a boil over medium-high heat and cook for 15 minutes, uncovered. Add the millet, reduce heat to low, and simmer for 30 minutes, covered. Stir in the coconut milk and green beans and cook for another 10 minutes over low heat, covered.

Remove from heat and season with the lemon juice and salt, to taste.

Serve hot or store in the fridge for up to 5 days, or freeze in zip-tight plastic bags or glass mason jars for up to 3 months.

ACCEPTING (AND CELEBRATING)
YOUR POSTPARTUM BODY

When you have a baby, your life transforms—and so does your body. In the first days after your little one's arrival, you'll probably be hyper-focused on the immediate healing at hand. Things you once took for granted, like walking and pooping, may now feel like climbing Everest. Take it moment by moment, move slowly and deliberately, and the pain *will* subside.

Once your acute aches begin to fade and the new baby buzz quiets to a hum, you may find the space to take in your body for the first time. You could discover that you're standing in a body that doesn't quite look like yours anymore, that things have changed. Physically, you have gone through a major metamorphosis—the biggest of your life. While you were pregnant, your body shifted and expanded to hold your growing baby. Your organs were pushed to the side as the fetus grew; your hips and thighs took on extra weight to help sustain baby; and your breasts expanded to new—and dazzling, if you are usually smaller chested—cup sizes.

Now, after birth, your body is between two states—it is no longer on loan to a small human being, but it's not as tight and strong as it once was. In the first forty days universe, this is the moment when we begin to embrace the understanding that there is no going back. The reality is that once your little one arrives, there are lots of things that have changed: You won't get your pre-baby sleep schedule back; you won't get your pre-baby social life back; and you won't get your pre-pregnancy body back. There is no going back; from here on out, there is only forward.

But, how exactly do you move forward if the image that shows up when you stand naked in front of the mirror is one that you don't enjoy at all? With tenderness and acceptance, for starters. And reverence right after that. You may be staring down unsightly stretch marks, a squishy, pouchy stomach, and underarm flab, but your job is to treat yourself with the same kindness and love that you give to your baby. In the beginning, this level of self-love requires *lots* of practice, but it does get easier, promise. The practice is built around a one-two punch of honor and acceptance. The honor, or the reverence, is for the miraculous project that your body just completed. You may have had a bit of help in the early stages and some guidance at the end, but you essentially made a human being and delivered her to the world—alone. This process utilized key components of your physical self: your blood and oxygen to grow and sustain the baby; your muscles and bones to hold you both up throughout the gestation period; your fat to store nutrients and prepare for breastfeeding. To accommodate your growing baby, your body was required to change. You will leave some of these changes behind after you give birth, but others will accompany you into parenthood. Even the women who count themselves among the small percentage who gained little weight during pregnancy or lost all of their baby weight within the first few months after giving birth will discover that their bodies are not exactly as they remember them. Their belly buttons are now raised slightly or sinking slightly, or one breast is permanently bigger than the other. Or maybe their skin is drier than it was before baby, or their feet are wider.

Here's where acceptance comes in, sliding in right behind the reverence for all that beautiful baby making you've just done. Accepting yourself as you are is the antidote to the shame you may feel when you see aspects of your maternal body that you're just not crazy about. When you accept yourself exactly as you are right now—with dark circles under your eyes and engorged breasts and mushy belly—you remain whole instead of picked apart, your various body parts shunted into categories of imperfection. When you're whole, you are stronger, and when you are stronger you're a more capable, available mother and partner. And most partners will admit that they find the mother of their child incredibly sexy after she gives birth—not just because of her curves, but because she had his (or her) baby.

But acceptance doesn't mean that you give up on regaining your strength and finding your center again. Once you've accepted that things are indeed different and have abandoned the notion of getting back to someplace you were before you had a baby, you can begin to set your sights on what it will feel like to move forward, to feel good in your skin again. It helps to stay away from Photoshopped images of supermodel mothers with their biologically impossible washboard abs. Instead, if you feel anxious to ignite some renewed vitality in your body, begin by turning to your center. I often suggest postpartum belly wrapping, also called rebozo, to bring new energy to a mother's center. Belly wrapping is used in many cultures throughout West Africa, Latin America, and Asia and is an effective way to reconnect the abdominal muscles that separated during birth and to support the lower back. You can use a long cloth to wrap yourself or use a Physiomat belt, which wraps around your belly and can be worn under clothing. (A quick Google search will lead you to instructional belly-wrapping videos, and the Physiomat belt can be ordered from Amazon.) The firm belly hug of a good wrap can feel delightful. But remember, belly binding is not about shrinking your middle. It's about bringing strength and energy to an area of the body that has been weakened by the effort of pregnancy and childbirth.

Place your loving hands on your belly and body and gently bring your awareness to your womb and vagina at least once every day. Tune in to how they feel. They have done hard work! Breathe into them and allow any feelings that come up to flow. It is essential that you connect with them consciously and regularly in the recovery phase—even more so if there were complications during birth—because this will initiate deep self-healing.

—ULRIKE REMLEIN, CHILDBIRTH EDUCATOR, DOULA, AND RED TENT FACILITATOR, NATISBON, GERMANY

congee

A bowl of congee is one of the most reassuring meals you can eat. In China and other Asian countries, this rice porridge is what you get served when you're a little under the weather. Soft, warm, and mushy, requiring minimal effort to digest, congee in its basic form is gentle and nurturing, the perfect food for a woman's body after birthing her child.

It also balances her tired-but-wired mental state. The mother's senses are taking in a million new bits of information, while simultaneously recovering from birth and processing change on every level. Creamy, white congee is wonderfully neutral; it's a relief just to taste it! It fills your belly in a clean, calm way, and making it doesn't require creativity or thought.

It also offers a fantastic blank canvas on which to improvise. Congee blows open whatever idea you had of porridge in the past. It welcomes all kinds of ingredients; take one big pot of congee and play with proteins, vegetables, and condiments, to eat it a different way each day. A little like risotto, congee can be made with broth instead of water—but without risotto's wine or cheese—then customized with whatever savory ingredients you have in the fridge. Or it can be turned into a dreamy rice pudding, swirled with stewed fruits and cream.

The power of congee is that it's such easy eating. It's a food that you (or a loved one) can make in your pj's after a long night rocking baby. Or scoop out a serving as a midnight snack; it is so gentle on the digestion, and so settling with its starches, it can help you slip more easily into brief hours of sleep. The ingredients are few, and should be there in your pantry—if you stocked up on provisions in the Gathering. And while it's simple enough to make on the stovetop, it can also be set to cook overnight in a slow cooker, ensuring that everyone in your home wakes up to a one-pot-meal that is infinitely pleasing to the palate and the belly.

WHITE RICE CONGEE

CONGEE IS PRESCRIBED ANY TIME that spleen *chi*—the energy that propels digestion and production of blood—needs to be replenished. It is a food of rebirth; its simplicity and clean taste feel so comforting in a weary or recovering body. One cup (210 g) of sticky rice (also called glutinous rice) is the secret to its nurturing texture—though if that grain is hard to find, use 3½ cups (665 g) white jasmine rice instead. Congee loves water, so if you sense it is getting too dried out, add another cup of water to the pot, stir, and continue to cook.

Serves 4–6 (plenty to store and use for days)

1½ cups (285 g) white jasmine rice
½ cup (105 g) white sticky rice

There are a few different methods for making congee (like a choose-your-own-congee-adventure book). Start each option by rinsing the rice several times in water, covering the rice with water, then swirling it around, then draining and repeating several times until the water runs clear when you drain it.

Option 1. Cook the rice in a rice cooker, as per instructions, so you end up with 4 to 4½ cups (780 to 875 g) cooked rice. The cooked rice will then go into a pot with 1 quart (960 ml) water. Over medium heat, bring to a boil then lower heat and cook for 45 minutes, covered, stirring often, checking to make sure the water level is always at least ½ inch (12 mm) above the rice level. Cook until the rice opens and softens. (If I remember to do it the night before, I like to soak my rice overnight, covered in water, before cooking it.)

Option 2. Another way to cook congee is on the stovetop. In a medium pot, bring the uncooked rice with 1 quart (960 ml) water, or enough water to cover the rice by 1½ inches (4 cm), to a boil over high heat. When it comes to a boil, reduce heat to a simmer and cook for 45 minutes, until the grains soften and open. You'll want to stir often and keep checking and adding water if it's been absorbed. Adding the sticky rice gives it an extra-full texture.

It's ready to eat hot. Store leftovers in the fridge for up to 5 days, or freeze in 3-cup (585-g) portions in 1-quart (960-ml) zip-tight plastic bags for up to 3 months.

RECIPE CONTINUED ON PAGE 156

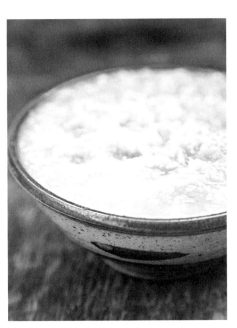

White Rice Congee

RECIPE CONTINUED FROM PAGE 155

VARIATION: **Chicken Ginger Congee**
To create a really flavorful congee and as a great way to use up leftovers, you can use 1 quart (960 ml) Chicken, Red Dates & Ginger Soup (page 138), or just 2 cups (480 ml) of the soup plus 2 cups (480 ml) water, in place of the 1 quart (960 ml) water in the basic White Rice Congee.

VARIATION: **Sweet Rice Congee with Black Sesame Seed Paste**
For a sweet treat, scoop 2 cups (390 g) of hot White Rice Congee into a bowl. Sprinkle with brown sugar or drizzle in some raw honey along with ground cinnamon, raisins, or, for a more decadent flourish, dried figs. You could also crack an egg or two into the congee while it's still cooking and swirl it in for a custardy effect that also adds protein. With or without the egg, I definitely recommend spooning in the Homemade Black Sesame Paste (see next column). Black sesame supports kidney energy—essential for reproductive health—and the paste is like a sweet, dark tahini.

TIP: *Congee leftovers can stretch in a million ways. Use them as a base under a stew, as a side dish with a splash of Bragg for flavor, or mix in some eggs and turn the congee into tasty fried rice patties.*

Black Sesame Seed Paste

THIS CAN BE USED AS a dip or spread with anything you like, as well as swirled into your rice congee.

Makes 1 cup (225 g)

1 cup (115 g) black sesame seeds
2 tablespoons honey
7 tablespoons (105 ml) olive oil or melted coconut oil

Blend everything together in a blender or food processor. This will take a little patience as you'll need to occasionally stop and push the seeds (with a wooden spoon or spatula—never with your hands) toward the blade and then return to blending. Keep going until you have a soft paste.

Store in a glass container in the fridge for up to 5 days. If it hardens in the fridge, you can spoon some out and warm it in a pan on the stovetop, adding a little more oil to soften it.

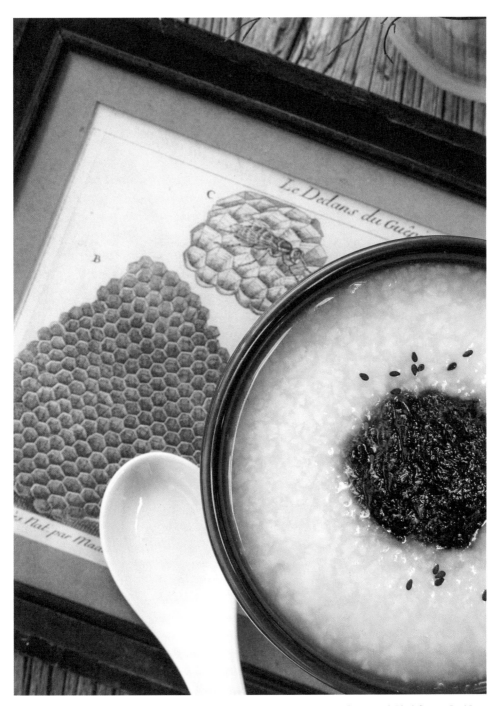

Sweet Rice Congee with Black Sesame Seed Paste

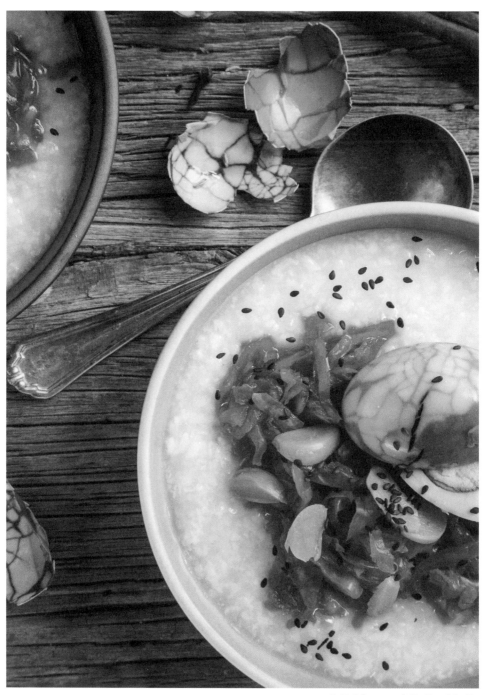

Pickled Congee with Tea Eggs & Pickles

PICKLED CONGEE WITH TEA EGGS & PICKLES

IN CHINA, tea eggs are traditionally eaten during the New Year and other special occasions and shared as symbols of fertility, health, prosperity, and wealth. What better time to enjoy them than after the arrival of your child! They are such a refreshingly surprising twist on the trusty hard-boiled egg. Store them in the fridge in their fragrant sauce of black tea, soy, sugar, and spice, then slice them onto steaming congee (or just grab a couple any time you need a protein boost). Tangy, salty pickles provide a superb contrast in this very flavorful congee mix.

Serves 4–6

4 cups (780 g) White Rice Congee (see page 155)

For the tea eggs:

12 large pasture-raised eggs

6 tablespoons (90 ml) soy sauce, tamari, or Bragg Liquid Aminos

2 teaspoons brown sugar or coconut sugar

1½ teaspoons Chinese five-spice powder

2 bags black tea

Optional toppings: sauerkraut, kimchee, pickles, minced green onion, extra soy sauce, watercress, chopped peanuts

Carefully put the eggs in a medium pot and add cold water to cover them by 1 inch (2.5 cm). Bring the water to a boil over high heat. Reduce heat to medium high and keep at a rolling boil for 8 to 10 minutes, then remove from heat.

Spoon the hard-boiled eggs into a bowl and rinse under cold water. (Do not discard the hot water.) Now roll the eggs gently on a flat surface to create light cracks across each egg, leaving the shells on and intact. (If there are kids around, they'll love this step!)

Return the eggs to the original pot of hot water and add the soy sauce, brown sugar, five-spice powder, and the tea bags. Bring everything to a quick boil over medium heat, and once boiling, lower heat and simmer for 40 minutes, covered. Turn off heat and let the eggs marinate in the sauce for up to 6 hours at room temperature (or if you're making these in advance, they can marinate in the fridge for up to 2 days). You can keep the eggs in the sauce in the fridge until you are ready to eat them, but they are best served warmed up or at room temperature.

To serve the tea eggs with the congee, add 2 cups (390 g) of cooked congee for 1 serving to a small pot (or use freshly made hot congee of your choice), adding enough water to cover the congee by ½ inch (12 mm). Stir, uncovered, over medium-low heat, until the congee is heated through and the added liquid is incorporated. Scoop the congee into your serving bowl and enjoy with the tea eggs and their savory sauce plus whatever optional toppings you like.

You can also add the peeled eggs and their sauce to other cooked grain dishes, or just warm them in a pan and eat them by themselves. These are great snacks to munch on during the day for some unique and tasty protein.

TIP: *If you can't find five-spice powder at your supermarket, there are recipes online for this blend containing star anise, fennel, black pepper, cinnamon, and cloves.*

BASIL & BEEF STRIPS CONGEE

ONE NIGHT I SERVED A mom-friend a bowl of congee with leftover grilled Thai beef salad from dinner the night before. The combination of tender meat, fragrant basil, and creamy rice was so delicious, it spawned this fusion dish, which benefits from the herb's immune-boosting, anti-inflammatory, and magnesium-rich properties. It will be especially loved by hungry menfolk in your home who may be craving a good steak.

Serves 4–6

For the brown rice congee:

1 cup (190 g) short-grain brown rice

½ cup (100 g) white rice

½ cup (105 g) white sticky rice

3 tablespoons sesame oil

1 clove garlic, peeled and finely chopped

1 cup (110 g) thinly sliced white or yellow onion

Pinch of sea salt

1 fresh chili pepper, seeds removed, minced (optional, if you want some heat)

1 tablespoon granulated cane or coconut sugar

½ cup (120 ml) soy sauce, tamari, or Bragg Liquid Aminos

1 pound (455 g) beef (cut of your choice), cut into thin strips, any length you like

½ cup (20 g) roughly chopped fresh basil leaves

Squeeze of fresh lime juice

To make the brown rice congee: In a medium pot, combine the short-grain brown rice, white rice, and sticky rice. Rinse it several times in water to get rid of excess starch, covering the rice with water, then swirling it around, then draining and repeating several times until the water runs clear when you drain it.

Add 3 cups (720 ml) water to the pot and bring to a gentle boil over medium-low heat. Reduce the heat to a simmer and cook until the rice opens and softens, keeping the pot half covered. Watch to make sure it does not boil over, stirring occasionally and checking to make sure the water level is always at least ½ inch (12 mm) above the rice level. This will take a minimum of 1 hour.

Meanwhile, heat 2 tablespoons of the sesame oil in a medium frying pan over medium-high heat. When the oil is hot, add the garlic, onion, salt, and chili pepper, if using, and cook over medium heat for 5 minutes, stirring frequently (and watching carefully) to make sure the garlic does not burn. Cook until the onions are soft but remove from the heat if they begin to get brown.

Once the oil is flavored with the garlic and chili pepper, you can add the sugar, soy sauce, and then the beef strips for a flash-fry, cooking over medium heat until the beef is to your liking. (I tend to like mine a little pink inside and tender.) Add the basil leaves and let it all simmer together over low heat for another 5 to 7 minutes, uncovered. This gives you a lovely sauce to pour over your congee. Finish with the squeeze of lime juice.

Turn off the heat and serve warm. Leftovers will keep for several days in the fridge.

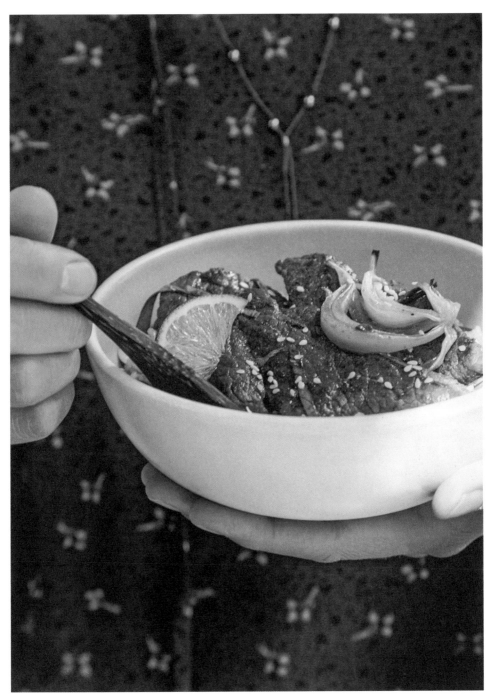

Basil & Beef Strips Congee

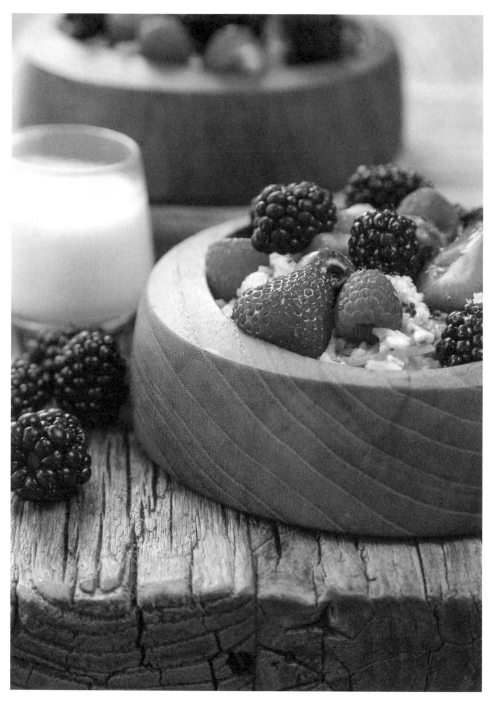

Oats & Chia Congee

OATS & CHIA CONGEE

THIS VERSION OF CONGEE REQUIRES no translation: It's oat porridge with a twist. Everyone in the family can dig in—oats deliver excellent nutrition and energy and fortify mom's lactation. Chia adds an extra protein kick. To make it extra easy to digest and to cut a few minutes off the cooking time, soak the oats in water for a few hours, or overnight, with a little squeeze of lemon juice and a pinch of salt.

Serves 6

2 cups (180 g) rolled oats

1½ cup (235 g) steel-cut oats

1-inch (2.5-cm) knob of fresh ginger, peeled and halved

Pinch of sea salt

¼ cup (40 g) chia seeds

½ cup (50 g) quinoa flakes (optional; add another ½ cup/120 ml water if using)

For the toppings:

1 cup (240 ml) milk (or cream, coconut milk, or nut milk of your choice)

2 tablespoons coconut oil or butter

¼ cup (60 ml) maple syrup, or to taste

Fresh or frozen fruit or berries, for serving (optional)

Chopped almonds or other nuts, for serving (optional)

In a medium pot, bring 4½ cups (1 L) water to a boil over medium-high heat. Add the rolled and steel-cut oats, the ginger, and salt. Reduce the heat to medium and let cook—three-quarters of the way covered—for 10 minutes, then reduce the heat to low and simmer for another 15 minutes; add more water if needed, keeping an eye on the pot so it doesn't boil over. Add the chia seeds and quinoa flakes, if using, during the last 15 minutes of cooking, stirring occasionally so the seeds and flakes separate and incorporate into the mixture. Once the grains are soft and creamy, and most of the liquid is absorbed, remove from heat.

When you are ready to eat, serve warm with the milk, coconut oil or butter, maple syrup to taste, plus fresh fruit and almonds, if you like.

Portion-freezing option: After the congee is cooked (and the chia seeds and quinoa have been added), let it cool on the stovetop. Spray muffin tins with cooking spray. Portion the congee into ½ cup (115 g) servings in the cups of the muffin tin. Flash-freeze for 4 to 5 hours, or until firm. Twist or tap out each serving and place them in large zip-tight plastic bags. When you are ready to eat, add one or two to a saucepan with some milk or water and reheat over low heat for 3 to 4 minutes, uncovered.

PINK CRANBERRY PORRIDGE

EATING COLORFUL FOOD TICKLES THE soul—it's a bit like applying a sweep of vivid lipstick. This bright pink bowl of farina gets its mood-lifting hue from tart cranberries that also add an unexpected flavor burst. It's extra good with a swirl of maple syrup—the combo brings to mind cozy autumn flavors and scents. If you're gluten-free, substitute quinoa flakes, or adapt this recipe to the Oats and Chia Congee (see previous page), using gluten-free oats.

Serves 4

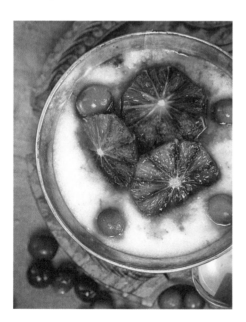

Pink Cranberry Porridge

1½ cups (145 g) frozen or fresh cranberries

Pinch of sea salt

¼ cup (55 g) granulated sugar or sweetener of your choice

¾ cup (130 g) farina

½ cup (120 ml) almond or coconut milk, for serving

Optional toppings: almonds, fresh sliced fruits, dried shredded coconut, bee pollen, or a drizzle of maple syrup or honey

In a medium pot, bring 2 cups (480 ml) water to a boil over high heat, add the cranberries and cook, uncovered, for 5 minutes, or until the cranberries pop and open. Add the salt and sugar and lower heat to a simmer. Whisk in the farina, stirring constantly for about 10 minutes over low heat, until it cooks into a light, fluffy, soft porridge. (You can add up to 1 cup/240 ml water, if needed, to keep the porridge light and airy.)

Turn off the heat and scoop the desired amount into your serving bowl. Whisk a few times to keep the porridge fluffy and swirl in the milk and whatever toppings you choose.

Store leftovers for up to 3 days in the fridge. Just remember to whisk the porridge a bit before adding your milk and toppings (and again after adding them, if you like).

THE FANTASY VISITOR

Who doesn't want to meet a brand-new baby? The impact of a baby's entrance into the world ripples out way beyond the child's immediate family and you may find yourself fielding requests from neighbors, extended family, friends, and colleagues wanting to experience the wonder that is this brand-new human being curled in your arms.

Be judicious with who gets to enter your haven. Many well-meaning visitors—even close family like grandparents and siblings—can unintentionally neglect to put your needs at the forefront and forget that a visit to your home may actually create *more* work for you. Most people don't, in fact, realize how precious a new mother's energy is during the early days home with baby and that simple acts like getting out of bed or making light conversation can be quite draining. Consider how, after delivery, you will be in an extremely vulnerable space, and it is wise to receive visitors who understand where you are and who will approach you gently, slowly, and quietly. Even close family members may have to wait to meet baby if you are not feeling up to the visit. Postpartum is your time to exert some very real self-care policies for yourself. Do what feels right!

In the spirit of encouraging all mothers to ask for what they need, here is some playful guidance for visitors-to-be that is gathered from some of MotherBees' postpartum doula colleagues. Feel free to share it smilingly with those who love you.

THE FIRST FORTY DAYS FANTASY VISITOR. . .
Learns that you are home alone with your baby because your partner has gone back to work (or for any other reason). She calls to ask if she can stop by later that day or the next day to spend a bit of time with you and bring you some food.

She knows that when she arrives at your home there may be a note on the door that says, "I'm napping. You can leave food at the door. I'll call you when I can." She doesn't take it personally and is happy you're getting some rest.

If you are open to a visit, she immediately puts the food she's made in the fridge—a large quantity that can be eaten with one hand, the leftovers frozen—gives you a hug, looks you in the eye, and asks, "how *are* you?" While you're answering she goes over to the sink saying, "I'm listening, I just need to wash my hands so I can hold the baby and give your arms a little break."

WHILE SHE IS AT THE SINK, SHE WASHES ALL OF YOUR DISHES.
After she washes the dishes, she takes baby only if he is fussy or you truly want a break—the fantasy visitor never interrupts mother-and-baby bonding. She then turns to you and asks, "How have the past week(s) been? What's been going really well for you? What's been hard for you?" The fantasy visitor doesn't try to instruct, change, or convince you about anything. She has confidence in your skills as a mother and is there to listen.

SHE DOESN'T STAY TOO LONG. THE FANTASY VISIT LASTS FOR FORTY-FIVE MINUTES TO AN HOUR.
The fantasy visitor does not expect to be hosted or doted on. She does not expect her needs to be met. She has come to your home because she is excited to take care of you—and to meet the new addition to your family!

ADZUKI & SWEET POTATO CONGEE

WITH ITS TRIO OF BEANS, root vegetable, and rice, this gentle congee makes good use of your stocked-up pantry. It uses the mildly sweet and fiber-rich adzuki bean, a food that's said to uplift the heart and that is used in many Chinese desserts. This congee's gingery taste can get enhanced with other spices, if you like—a touch of chili powder and smoked sea salt is one of my favorite twists.

Serves 6

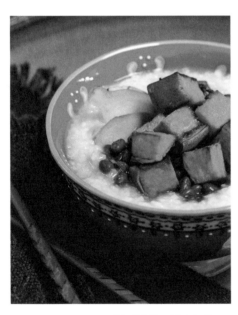

Adzuki & Sweet Potato Congee

5 cups (975 g) White Rice Congee (see page 155)

1 cup (135 g) peeled and cubed sweet potato or yam

1 cup (170 g) canned organic adzuki beans

5 tablespoons (75 g) brown cane sugar (or raw honey or other sweetener of your choice)

2-inch (5-cm) knob of fresh ginger, peeled, mashed, and minced (you want as much juice in the dish as possible so do this over a small bowl)

Pinch of sea salt (optional)

In a medium pot over low heat, combine the congee with 6 cups (1.4 L) cold water (or enough to cover the congee by ½ inch/ 12 mm). Add the sweet potatoes, beans, sugar, and ginger juice (and any little soft bits you may want), and the salt, if using. Cook, three-quarters of the way covered, for 40 minutes, stirring occasionally. Keep an eye on the water level and add more cold water to prevent sticking if needed.

Store leftovers in the fridge for up to 5 days, or freeze in 1-quart (960-ml) zip-tight plastic bags in 3-cup (675-g) portions for up to 3 months.

mother's bowls

When life as you knew it before has changed irrevocably and everything is suddenly new—your body, your family, and this sweet little person in your arms—you won't care about eating the same thing on repeat if it's healthy, tasty, and fresh. Just a few minor variations will keep it interesting. That's the thinking behind my Mother's Bowls. They let you rotate through a few components—protein, greens, whole grains, or root vegetables—and mix and match them as you see fit. It's a postpartum survival strategy; your rations are lined up for the mission ahead and when you open the fridge door, you'll emit a joyful cry, "Thank God! There's something to eat!"

These bowls were inspired by an experience I had while getting lost in the back streets of Tokyo. Confused and disoriented, I stumbled into a restaurant looking for help. Soon, I was serving myself lunch. At this eatery, the cooks—a team of women—put out a Japanese smorgasbord of earthy, hearty foods, simply and deliciously cooked, and let patrons create their own servings in big, wooden bowls. In Eastern cultures, root vegetables are seen as grounding, and sweet, earthy tastes of well-prepared grains can be grounding and comforting, too. My custom-made serving of squash, vegetables, homemade tofu, and seaweed left me utterly calmed and strengthened, as if I'd been picked up and given a hug. It was only as I left the restaurant that I saw the name: Mothers! How fitting.

What follows is a system for ensuring that you and your immediate family eat well on very busy days. Make one or two things from each food group in advance—or have a helper prep them—then store in glass containers in the fridge for three days at a time. When you're hungry, scoop out a combo of three or more things using grains or root vegetables as a solid base on which to place your proteins and lighter vegetables. Then, warm it up a little (or let it get up to room temperature, at least), adorn with toppings, and add drizzles of raw oils as you see fit.

Let your eyes guide your hand. The fun part of throwing a bowl together is that it can be a little art piece. Splash some purple or crimson on your greens in the form of sauerkraut or kimchi and make patterns of seaweed shreds or even popcorn. Notice how the parts come together: The invigorating sourness of the kraut or splash of vinegar against the earthy sweetness of the squash, and the crunch of seeds against rich and smooth avocado is not only fun, it's an exercise in balancing flavors, textures, and colors in one dish—a time-honored wellness practice said to balance the body and mind. To get you started, I include my favorite bowl combinations that take inspiration from points around the globe. I'm sure you'll soon come up with many more.

Turn to one of these bowls on a day that you feel scattered or jittery, anxious or irritated. The sustaining power of protein, the rooting effect of root vegetables, the brain-calming effect of fats are grounding. This meal will help you stand in your role as the pillar of the family, baby in your arms and your feet on terra firma.

Group 1: **GRAINS**

(if you don't eat grains, use root vegetables instead)

- Rice (brown, black, red, purple, wild, sticky, white, jasmine, basmati)

- Quinoa

- Millet

- Amaranth

- Barley

- Buckwheat

- Polenta (cooked from scratch, or you can buy logs of precooked polenta)

- Oats (steel-cut, rolled, quick)

- Wheat berries or bulgur

- Couscous or Israeli couscous (larger pearls)

- Pasta (fresh, frozen, dried. . . whatever is convenient; think noodles, spaghetti, gnocchi, ramen; if you aren't eating gluten, you can find buckwheat, corn, spelt, quinoa, bean, even sweet potato pasta)

Group 2: **PROTEINS**

- Eggs (scrambled, poached, hard-boiled, over-easy, fried)

- Chicken (poached, roasted, cut up, pan-fried)

- Pork (shredded, pulled, bacon)

- Beef (ground, stew pieces, strips of cooked steak/flank, oxtail pieces)

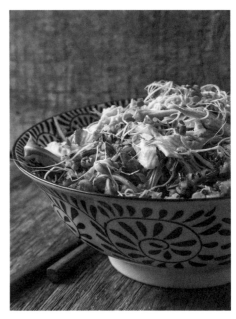

Asian Bowl

- Bison (ground is most often how you see it)

- Lamb (ground or strips of cooked flank)

- Fish (cooked, pickled, smoked); shellfish like scallops, crabs, shrimp, mussels; things in a tin or can that are easy to add to anything like sardines, mackerel, herring; breaded and pan-fried tiny fish like smelt or larger fillets like halibut or salmon or bass)

- Legumes (green lentils, adzuki beans, cannellini beans, pinto beans, garbanzo beans)

- Meatballs (from any ground meat)

Group 3: VEGETABLES

- Roasted (carrots, parsnips, fingerling potatoes, yams, sweet potatoes, winter squash, onions, beets)
- Pan-fried (Swiss chard, kale, bok choy, spinach, caramelized onions, leeks, shallots, red and green cabbage)
- Steamed (carrots, celery, string beans, asparagus, broccoli, cauliflower)
- Grated (carrots, parsnips, celery root)
- Mashed (yams, sweet potatoes, winter squash, celery root, parsnips)

Group 4: TOPPINGS

- Avocado
- Soy sauce, tamari, Bragg Liquid Aminos, or coconut aminos (they are delicious and soy free!)
- Nutritional yeast
- Sesame seeds
- Flaxseeds
- Hemp seeds
- Sunflower seeds
- Nuts (almonds, cashews, hazelnuts, pistachios, peanuts, macadamia, pine nuts, walnuts; raw or dry roasted—try to avoid oil roasted and heavily salted)
- Oils (flax, avocado, coconut, walnut, sesame)
- Melted butter (grass-fed)
- Olives (green, black)
- Herbs and spices (chili powder, a dash of cayenne, minced basil leaves, sea salt, fresh ground pepper, paprika, minced dill, et cetera)

Here are some combinations I like:

#1 ASIAN BOWL

IN A MEDIUM FRYING PAN, over medium-low heat, combine the following and heat until warm:

Leftover congee (whatever type you have)
Fresh greens (arugula, chard, kale, spinach)
Pan-fried or oven-baked bacon or sausage pieces
Chili powder (optional)

Season with the chili powder if you want some extra heat and if that matches the leftover congee you're using. Transfer to a bowl and eat warm.

#2 HEARTY AUTUMN BOWL

IN A SINGLE-SERVING BOWL, combine the following:

Roasted winter squash or sweet potatoes
Kale or any dark leafy green vegetable of a hearty nature sautéed in butter
Pan-fried bacon strips

Top with a drizzle of maple syrup and a handful of toasted pumpkin seeds. Eat warm.

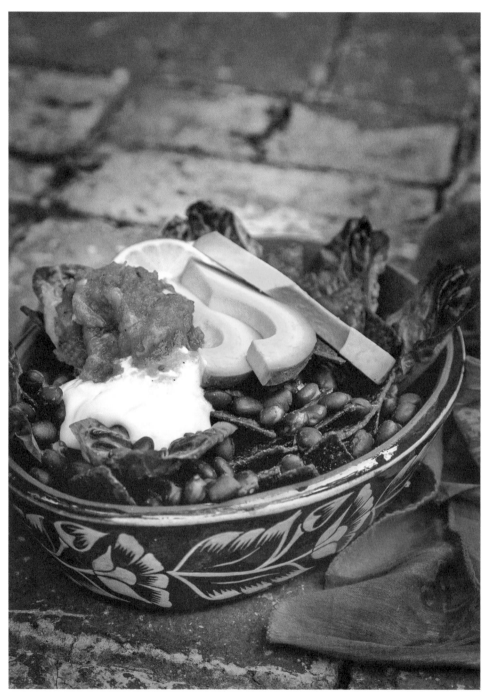

Mexican Bowl

#3 SCANDINAVIAN BOWL

IN A SERVING BOWL, LAYER the following ingredients:

Cooked wild rice

A few canned or jarred herring, mackerel, or sardines

A halved or chopped-up hard-boiled egg

A spoonful or two of mayo

Boiled new potatoes (optional)

Pickles and paprika (optional)

This Nordic-inspired meal can be eaten cold or the rice can be warmed with the oily fish in a frying pan, then transferred to the bowl.

#4 ITALIAN BOWL

IN A MEDIUM BOWL, ADD the following for a warming, comforting pasta bowl:

Cooked noodles of your choice, either with gluten or gluten-free (rice, bean, corn, or buckwheat noodles are all great options); warmed pasta sauce (add mushrooms and onions and arugula or chard for a heartier sauce)

Meatballs (easy to make; just combine the ground meat of your choice with an egg or two and any other herbs or spices you like, such as basil or cumin, and season with salt and pepper, then cook)

#5 FRENCH BOWL

IN A BOWL LAYER THESE together:

Leftover (or freshly cooked) risotto

Pieces of whole roasted fish (or pan-fried fish fillet)

Onion pieces sautéed in some butter until deep golden and very flavorful

1 squeeze of fresh lemon juice

Slices of a yummy French cheese (which will melt over the warmed risotto and fish) and sourdough baguette pieces (quick "croutons," optional)

#6 MEXICAN BOWL

IN A BOWL LAYER THESE:

Leftover or freshly cooked beans (any kind you want)

Shredded lettuce

Grated cheese (optional)

Leftover ground meat (any kind—beef, lamb, chicken, bison) or cook some up quickly in a pan until browned

Salsa

Avocado slices

For an extra layer and added crunch, feel free to add organic corn chips, and eat with your hands like nachos.

#7 INDIAN (CURRY) BOWL

IN A BOWL LAYER THE following:

Basmati rice or leftover cooked lentils

Curry powder or curry sauce (available in the international section of grocery stores)

Stir-fried or steamed vegetables and sliced ginger (carrots, peppers, broccoli, mushrooms, peas)

Toasted peanuts or cashews

the power foods

"Because it's good for you." In a few years, you'll almost certainly be saying this to your child, as you serve up something new. Right now, it's you who gets to hear this mother's mantra! An important piece of postpartum eating is food that works deeply on the depleted body, replenishing what's missing, and supports lactation, so that baby thrives and you feel vital as well. This food is completely fine to outsource: Get your partner or a friend to make it for you (most of these recipes are extremely fast and easy to prepare) and keep an open mind.

From the very light, but system-warming "first food" of Ginger Fried Rice (see page 175), traditionally served after birth, to lactation-inducing Fish, Papaya & Peanut Soup (see page 178), to heavy-hitter pig trotters, and rebuilding organ meats, these are the foods that your grandmother or mother-in-law would have cooked with her eyes closed. She would have made you consume them in order to rebuild your blood, boost your chi, or energy, enrich breast milk, and balance hormones and mood. And she would have made sure they tasted good! (How else would she ensure you got your fill?) This commitment to good taste has been captured here, with simple new recipes inspired by the old ways that I guarantee you will enjoy.

If you're already on board with nutrient-dense eating, nibbling a few bites of liver and kidney won't phase you. If the thought of organ meats gives you pause, however, consider that they have been revered as sacred foods throughout time in traditional cultures worldwide, especially in regards to childbearing. Easily prepared, they are nature's most potent source of vitamins, which pass on to baby in your milk. From the Chinese point of view, consuming organ meats from animals helps to support the correlating organs in us. Childbearing draws on our reserves of jing, or constitutional life essence, which is made and stored in the kidneys; eating kidney meat meets this lack, promoting longevity. Eating liver, meanwhile, supports our liver meridian, which is essential for the free flow of energy through the body.

The best argument for dipping into these dishes is that they are supplements on a fork. Just a few bites will help rebuild a body that has just finished building its greatest creation—a baby!—and will support you as you continue to give to others, day in and day out.

LIVER & GREENS

ANCIENT CHINA'S *Book of Rites*—A kind of guidebook to living a proper life—lists liver as one of the prized "eight delicacies" because it helps our bodies clear away the accumulation of toxins that can lead to depression and disease. In the West, liver is prized as a powerhouse of nutrients (vitamins A, B, D, and E, iron, and more) that are critical before, during, and after making a baby. Eating liver erases fatigue—the lift is palpable—and I always encourage pregnant women and lactating moms to take their liver once a week. Chicken liver is the mildest-tasting kind and fairly easy-to-source organic, which is important. This spicy twist on a classic dish turns this power food into a surprisingly light delicacy. Serve with warm rice.

Serves 2

3 organic chicken livers, sliced into strips (about ½ cup/115 g)

3 tablespoons cooking oil (avocado oil, coconut oil, or animal fat)

¼ of a white or yellow onion, thinly sliced

½ red pepper, seeds removed, thinly sliced

3 long, thin slices of peeled, fresh ginger (each about 2 inches/5 cm long)

2 tablespoons soy sauce, tamari, or Bragg Liquid Aminos

1 tablespoon sesame oil

2 loosely packed cups (40 g) organic baby spinach

Gently rinse the chicken livers under cold water and pat dry with a paper towel. Set aside on a plate.

In a hot pan, heat the cooking oil over high heat. When the oil is smoking a bit, add the onions and red pepper and sauté for 8 to 10 minutes, until the onions are golden brown. Add the ginger and cook for another 3 to 5 minutes, then add the livers, soy sauce, and sesame oil, and cook until the livers are barely brown. They will cook fast (in less than 5 minutes), so stir frequently and keep a close watch. Add the spinach and turn off the heat, covering the pan with a lid so it wilts, 3 to 5 minutes.

This dish is best eaten right when cooked, so serve immediately.

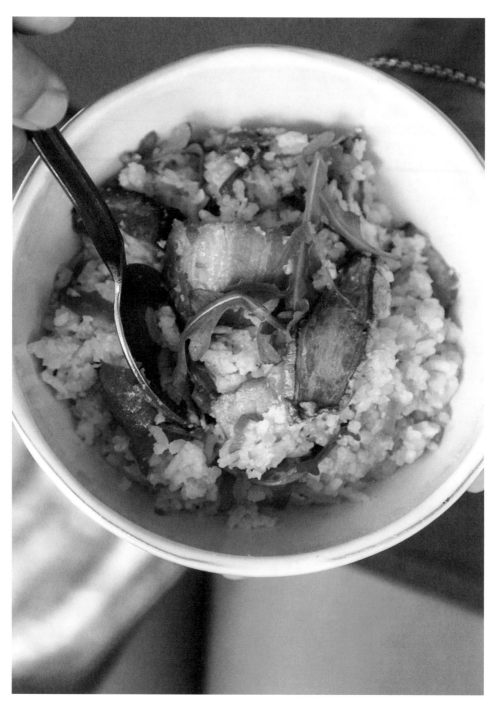

Ginger Fried Rice

GINGER FRIED RICE

IF A CHINESE ELDER WERE to visit you immediately after birth, this is likely the offering they'd bring. Light and warming, its star ingredient is ginger, to boost blood circulation and balance excess "wind" in the body after birth. Ginger Fried Rice travels well; it can be brought to you in containers and eaten at room temperature if there's no option to reheat. This is the dish that *anyone* can make for mom and that your other kids will enjoy as well. (Truth be told, it has a fun hint of Chinese takeout, just without any bad ingredients.) Weeks after baby comes, when everyone's found their groove, it will still be a go-to meal for mom that she can easily make herself.

Serves 2

2 cups (410 g) cooked white rice (leftover rice will work best here) or you can make it fresh (see directions next column)

3 tablespoons sesame oil, plus more as needed (see Tips, next column)

3 pieces of 2-inch (5 cm) bacon slices (optional)

2 cloves garlic, finely chopped

1 slice of fresh ginger, peeled and thinly sliced

2 large pasture-raised eggs, beaten with a pinch of sea salt

2 tablespoons thinly sliced green onion

Sea salt and freshly ground pepper

If making rice from scratch specifically for this dish: In a medium pot, wash and rinse 1 cup (185 g) white rice (any kind, short or long grain or jasmine, et cetera), several times until the cloudy water runs clear. Add 1 cup (240 ml) water with a pinch of sea salt and bring to a rapid boil over high heat. Add the rinsed rice, reduce heat, and cook, covered, until the rice is fluffy and the water is absorbed. A rice cooker will simplify the process significantly.

Using 2 cups of this rice, or leftover rice, proceed to fried rice directions: Heat the oil in a frying pan over medium-low heat, add bacon (if using), garlic, and fresh ginger, and cook until tender and fragrant. Add the cooked rice to the pan and spread it out evenly, making a thick layer, and cook, uncovered, over medium heat for 10 minutes, stirring occasionally.

Pour the beaten eggs into the rice and continue to stir frequently, until the eggs are cooked, about 5 minutes. Add the green onions and cook for another 2 minutes, uncovered, until the rice is golden in color and the eggs and onions are cooked. Season with salt and freshly ground pepper to taste. Serve warm.

TIPS: *I like to keep the rice fluffy. As you fry the rice, add more oil to the pan if necessary to keep it from drying out or sticking.*

It's easy to toss in a medley of vegetables like carrots, onions, peas, corn, broccoli, and mushrooms.

SLOW-BRAISED PIG TROTTERS

WHEN MY AUNT INITIATED ME into *zuo yuezi*, this tasty dish was her bribe to keep me tucked up in bed. I'd scoop the sauce out onto steaming rice, even after all the meat was gone from the pot. I didn't know then what its magic alchemy of ingredients was doing for me: The black vinegar was cleansing my blood, the ginger was dispelling wind, the brown sugar was chasing dampness, and the sesame was boosting circulation. It just tasted so good! A medley of sweet, sour, and salty tastes with a hit of crunchy texture, it is the ultimate harmony of flavors. Pig trotters—the meat from pigs' feet—sounds like extremely primitive fare, but consider them a gift from Mother Nature, rich in body-heating fat and healing gelatin, and a source of rich flavor when braised in liquid. You can find them at butchers and at Asian markets. Choose pasture-raised pork if you can get ahold of it.

Serves 6

2 tablespoons sesame oil

1-inch (2.5-cm) knob of fresh ginger, peeled and cut into thin slivers

1 trotter (pig's foot), cut into 1- to 2-inch (2.5- to 5-cm) chunks (you'll want to ask your butcher to do this for you)

1½ cups (360 ml) sweetened Chinese black vinegar or balsamic vinegar

¼ cup (55 g) packed brown sugar or coconut sugar

¼ cup (60 ml) soy sauce, tamari, or Bragg Liquid Aminos

4 hard-boiled pasture-raised eggs, peeled and left whole (optional)

White rice or congee (optional)

Heat the sesame oil in a medium braising pot over medium heat. Add the ginger slivers and cook for 8 to 10 minutes, stirring frequently, until they are dry and toasted on all sides and fragrant, watching carefully to make sure they don't burn. Remove from heat.

Meanwhile, in another medium pot, bring 3 cups (720 ml) water to a boil over high heat. Add the chopped trotter to the boiling water and blanch for 10 minutes, covered. Drain the trotter, rinse under cold water, and drain again.

To the braising pot with the cooked ginger slices, add the blanched trotter, vinegar, brown sugar, soy sauce, and ½ cup (120 ml) water, or enough to cover the trotter by ½ inch (12 mm).

Bring everything to a quick boil, then reduce the heat to low and simmer for 45 minutes, covered. In the last 15 minutes, you can add the pre-peeled hard-boiled eggs, if you're using them.

The dish is ready once the sauce has turned thick and the trotter is soft and fully browned. The skin will often start breaking apart when it's ready. Serve immediately, or keep the trotter in its sauce in the fridge for up to 5 days. Enjoy!

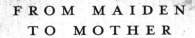

FROM MAIDEN TO MOTHER

Though countless women have done it before you and countless will do it after you, becoming a mother is a big deal. A very big deal. You have not only created a life, but you have moved through one of the biggest initiations of your *own* life.

Certain spiritual traditions believe that a woman will go through three stages in her lifetime: maiden, mother, and crone (a term that may have a negative connotation in modern society, but actually represents a powerful woman emanating the radiance of a lifetime of accumulated wisdom). Each stage is marked by a rite of passage: menstruating for the first time, giving birth to your first child, and, finally, menopause. Blood is the driving force behind each stage—the first blood of initial menstruation, the blood that naturally accompanies childbirth, and the cessation of bleeding at menstruation. The stages also correspond to the three lunar cycles: waxing moon, full moon, and waning moon.

The maiden is thought to be a young girl driven by curiosity and playfulness. She is exploring sexuality for the first time and is focused deeply on her own place in the world. As she grows into womanhood she will enter the next stage, mother, where she will experience the full expression of her capacity to nurture and be compassionate. Finally, she will transition into the crone stage, a period of life marked by wisdom and giving back to society.

The transitions from one stage to another are each significant initiations for a woman, as established ways of being fall away to reveal a land that has yet to be discovered. When a maiden becomes a mother she is required to reprioritize her universe, placing another being at the forefront of her attention—before her own feelings and desires. This shifting of her focus propels her forward into the next chapter of her life, where old systems are promptly dismantled and new methods must be created. Things don't look like they used to.

Traditional communities understand that a mother is a divine and powerful being. She is at the peak of her receptivity, full like the moon. She has a wide-open heart and is equipped with the ability to unconditionally love another. And while the early weeks of parenthood are a very real adjustment, she is designed to incorporate new ways of thinking and feeling, to entertain and even welcome a range of emotions and ideas.

And as you step fully into your role as mother, it's also important to acknowledge who you were before you gave birth as well as who you will be at the end of your childbearing years. All three of these pieces are in you, always. You can celebrate the new, mourn what has just ended, while also reveling in the traces that still exist.

FISH, PAPAYA & PEANUT SOUP

THIS LACTATION-BOOSTING SOUP IS THE second-most-famous postpartum dish in Chinese families, following pig trotters, which takes the number 1 spot. So many new moms report with wonder that this fragrant, simple soup seemed to turn up their milk flow; tradition says it's the mix of papaya juice, fish proteins, and peanuts that stimulates the milk ducts to release their bounty. Though it sounds exotic, it's actually a cinch to prepare. This is a great one to ask a favorite aunt (or friend) to make for you—let her shop for the fish and fruit and concoct it in her kitchen!

Serves 6–8

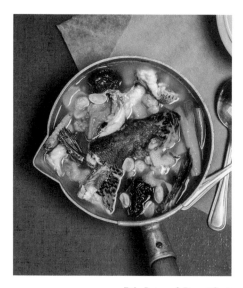

Fish, Papaya & Peanut Soup

Sea salt

1-inch (2.5-cm) knob of fresh ginger, peeled and cut into 6 thin slices

2 whole (head included) small fish or 1 medium fish (about 2 pounds/910 g total), such as black bass, tilapia, trout, or red snapper

½ of a medium papaya, peeled, seeded, and cut into medium cubes

2 tablespoons unsalted peanuts (keep the outer red skin on if you can)

2 whole green onion stalks, white ends trimmed off

3 medium tomatoes, halved, with seeds left in

4 Chinese red dates (optional; see "Pantry Resources," page 124)

In a medium pot over high heat, bring 2 quarts (2 L) water to a boil, then add a pinch of sea salt and the ginger.

Rinse the fish under cold water and add to the boiling water. Add the papaya, peanuts, green onions, tomatoes, and red dates, if using, reduce the heat, and simmer for 1 hour, covered.

Taste and add more salt, if needed. Strain the soup if you just want to drink the broth, or eat all the bits of fish, if you like, watching out for the bones.

Drink throughout the day. Store leftovers in the fridge for up to 2 days, or freeze in zip-tight bags or glass mason jars (see box, page 130) for up to 3 months.

BREADED GINGERED KIDNEYS (or Kidneys Dusted with Cornmeal and Ginger)

THIS IS MY ODE TO Auntie Ou and her legendary feat of eating one pig kidney each day throughout her postpartum period. Ginger, cornmeal, tamari or soy sauce, and a butter and broth sauce make this version comforting and almost luxurious in texture. I don't advise consuming kidneys daily, but taken once a week, a few bites of this traditional food will show your kidney organ system some love. This helps to replenish your energy at a deep-seated level and support your reproductive system, too, which is connected to the kidney system.

Serves 2

For the marinade:

1 tablespoon soy sauce, tamari, or Bragg Liquid Aminos

1 teaspoon brown sugar, coconut sugar, or honey

2-inch (5-cm) knob of fresh ginger, peeled and finely minced (or use a garlic press, which will press the pieces into juice)

2 tablespoons sake or white wine (optional)

1 teaspoon cooking oil (avocado, sesame, or melted coconut)

1 pair of pork or lamb kidneys, or 2 pairs of chicken kidneys (because they're smaller)

2 tablespoons sesame oil

1-inch (2.5-cm) knob of fresh ginger, peeled and minced

¼ cup (30 g) all-purpose flour or gluten-free flour of your choice

1 large pasture-raised egg, beaten

¼ teaspoon sea salt

¼ cup (45 g) cornmeal or blanched almond meal/flour

1 tablespoon black sesame seeds

Condiment options: lemon juice, Sriracha/ mayonnaise, miso/mayo, Chinese black vinegar/mayo, or mustard

To make the marinade, stir together all the ingredients in a bowl large enough to hold the kidneys.

Prepare the kidneys by cutting them in half horizontally. Remove the vein and rinse them under running water. Dry with a paper towel. Chop into bite-size pieces, then add them to the marinade. Let sit at room temperature for 15 to 30 minutes, then cover with plastic wrap and refrigerate.

RECIPE CONTINUED ON PAGE 180

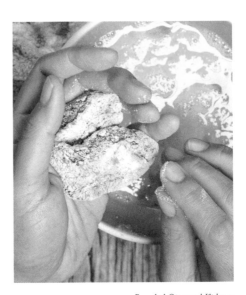

Breaded Gingered Kidneys

RECIPE CONTINUED FROM PAGE 179

When you're ready to eat, warm a pan with the sesame oil over medium heat. Add the ginger and cook until it softens and browns.

Meanwhile, arrange the flour, beaten egg, sea salt, cornmeal, and sesame seeds in separate bowls in a row on the counter. Drain the kidneys and dip them in the flour, egg, cornmeal, and sesame seeds to coat.

Add the breaded kidneys to the pan with the ginger and cook for 5 to 7 minutes, until they are golden brown and crispy on all sides (be careful not to overcook them).

Eat right away with your condiment of choice. The cornmeal and sesame seed dusting will mostly fall off, but mix it back in when you eat it, taking a bite of the crunchy bits along with some of the kidney. It's delicious.

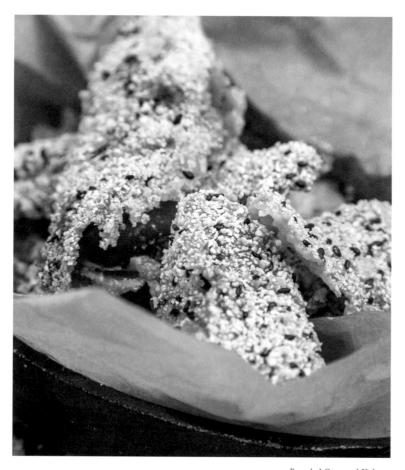

Breaded Gingered Kidneys

nut milks, seed milks
& smoothies

In India, a new mother will likely drink cup after cup of warm, fresh cow's milk with a scoop of ghee and a spoonful of honey to replenish her after birth. Always consumed warm, it's a fortifying and clarifying sattvic *or "peaceful" food, perfect for postpartum with its Ayurveda-approved qualities: sweet, soft, and pleasant. But I've found that women's digestive systems don't do as well on the version of cow's milk available in our Western supermarkets—invariably pasteurized, then typically served refrigerated, making it mucus forming, heavy and cold, stripped of many of the truly nourishing properties, and potentially irritating to mother's and baby's digestive systems.*

Instead, I turn to freshly made nut and seed milks that are enhanced with extra goodies like chia, dates, spices, and black sesame, in a fusion of old and new approaches from East and West. With their protein and fabulous raw fats, and clutch of important trace minerals, homemade nut milks deliver excellent nutrition in liquid form, ensuring you get a fast boost when you need it. They can be consumed at room temperature or heated up, with a dash of honey and vanilla if you like, for an extra-nurturing mug. And they're actually easier *to acquire than dairy milk, because if mom has squirreled away her pantry provisions, they can be made in her kitchen in just a few minutes with no grocery run necessary. Nut milks are the perfect food for a cozy hibernation period.*

If you love dairy milk and tolerate it well, any of these recipes can be customized to use whole-fat milk instead of nut milk. Using raw (unpasteurized) milk will be the most healing and nutritious option, with its bounty of intact proteins, enzymes, and protective factors, and delicious, full-cream taste—it should be consumed warm for digestibility, but keep your eye on the saucepan as high heat will destroy some of those delicate nutrients. Unpasteurized milk can be tough to find. Check out realmilk.com *to find sources listed by state.*

Another way to enjoy nut-based drinks is a hearty smoothie that uses coconut milk from a can— coconut is another traditional warming food—or mix coconut water with greens. Packed with greens or other great ingredients, these thick smoothies are such a treat, they put a huge smile on every mom who receives them—proof, it seems, that they're capturing that sattvic *effect!*

If you've never made nut milk before, you might envision it taking lots of work and gear. It doesn't. A decent-quality blender, a bowl, and cheesecloth or a nut milk bag and five minutes—of someone else's time, hopefully—will result in a drink that will make mother feel as blissful and satisfied as the baby who may be dozing, or drinking her own serving of milk at the breast.

CASHEW CHIA MILK

IN ANCIENT MAYAN CULTURE, TINY chia seeds were consumed for strength—a Western parallel to Eastern black sesame. They're easy to find today and fun to use in nut milks and smoothies for some added texture. They also add extra protein and good fatty acids, making this milk a delicious and satisfying snack.

Serves 4

4 cups (480 g) raw or dry-roasted cashews, unsalted

3 fresh dates, pits removed (optional)

2 tablespoons ground cinnamon

2 tablespoons pure vanilla extract (optional)

¼ cup (40 g) chia seeds, unsoaked

Put everything in a blender, then add 7 cups (1.7 L) water. Blend until the milk is frothy, 2 to 3 minutes.

Whatever straining method you're using (a nut milk bag, fine-mesh strainer, or cheesecloth), hold it over a large bowl and slowly pour the contents of the blender into it, letting all the milk drain into the bowl. You may need to do this in more than one batch depending on how much pulp you can hold in the strainer or bag. The leftover nut meal can be used for baking or compost, or freeze it for another occasion.

Drink right away or store in the fridge for 2 to 3 days.

BLACK ALMOND MILK

BLACK SESAME SEEDS ARE A staple of the traditional postpartum pantry because they support lactation, longevity, *and* beauty. They're *zuo yuezi*'s triple threat! Adding them to almond milk is one of my favorite ways to enjoy them, and a dollop of coconut milk will make the elixir extra creamy. For a sweet, perfumed addition that pairs perfectly with almonds and black sesame, add a few drops of rosewater; the result is very exotic and sensual.

Serves 4

4 cups (560 g) raw or dry-roasted almonds (see Tip, opposite page)

3 tablespoons black sesame seeds

Pinch of sea salt

1 teaspoon sweetener of your choice, such as honey, fresh dates, coconut sugar, organic maple syrup, organic stevia, or to taste

1 tablespoon full-fat coconut milk, coconut oil, or organic soy lecithin (whatever you have on hand to give the milk a thick and creamy texture; optional)

A few drops of rosewater for a slightly perfumed scent and taste (optional)

If using soaked almonds, drain them. Put everything in a blender, then add 7 cups (1.7 L) water. Blend until the milk is frothy, 2 to 3 minutes.

Whatever straining method you're using (a nut milk bag, fine-mesh strainer, or cheesecloth), hold it over a large bowl and slowly pour the contents of the blender into it, letting all the milk drain into the bowl.

You may need to do this in more than one batch depending on how much pulp you can hold in the strainer or bag. The leftover nut meal can be used in place of almond flour in your favorite gluten-free cookies, added to granola, or used in our Gooey Chocolate Brownies (page 205).

Pour the strained milk into a glass jar or pitcher. Serve immediately, straight up; use in tea or Ceremonial Hot Chocolate (page 216); or as a base for smoothies. Store the remainder in the fridge for 2 to 3 days.

TIP: *If you have the time, soaking the almonds in water overnight will make them easier to blend and more digestible, but this is an optional step.*

CHOCOLATE HAZELNUT MILK

HAZELNUTS, HEMP SEEDS, AND CACAO combine to make chocolate milk for grown-ups. This amazing triumvirate of super foods gives you raw cacao's energizing lift, along with hemp seeds' protein boost, and doesn't leave you with the crash that your coffee or latte would. Use it as a base for a smoothie or warm it up for an instant hot chocolate! You can buy ground flax meal or make it yourself by grinding whole flaxseeds (brown or golden) in a clean spice or coffee grinder. I keep two grinders at my home, one for coffee beans and one for spices and seeds.

Serves 4

4 cups (540 g) shelled hazelnuts

3 tablespoons hemp seeds

3 tablespoons flaxseed meal

3 tablespoons cacao powder or organic cocoa powder or carob

Pinch of sea salt

5 tablespoons (75 ml) honey

Place everything in a blender, then add 7 cups (1.7 L) water. Blend until the milk is frothy, 2 to 3 minutes.

Whatever straining method you're using (a nut milk bag, fine-mesh strainer, or cheesecloth), hold it over a large bowl and slowly pour the contents of the blender into it, letting all the milk drain into the bowl. You may need to do this in more than one batch depending on how much pulp you can hold in the strainer or bag. The leftover nut meal can be used for baking in a day or two if stored in the fridge, or you can compost it.

Delicious served right away. Refrigerate the rest in a glass jar or pitcher for up to 3 days.

TIP: *Dig into your bag of organic hemp seeds often, as they add a wonderful dash of protein and omega-3 fatty acids to both savory foods (congees and vegetables) and sweet ones (desserts and smoothies).*

AVOCADO, COCONUT & LIME SMOOTHIE

THIS IS A SMOOTHIE THAT is simultaneously refreshing and warming. Packed with good saturated fat for creamy, nourishing energy and lubricating oils, it gets a fresh twist with tangy lime. This is a perfect, easily digestible meal made of ingredients you most likely already have on hand. Along with fresh guacamole and my Chocolate Mousse (page 197), it makes a strong case for keeping a stash of avocados in the pantry.

Serves 2

½ avocado, pit removed, flesh scooped out of peel

2 cups (480 ml) light (not full-fat) coconut milk

2½ tablespoons honey

1 tablespoon lime juice

Pinch of sea salt

Shredded unsweetened coconut and/or lime zest for garnish (optional)

Put the avocado, coconut milk, honey, lime juice, and salt in a blender and blend until smooth. Top with the coconut and lime zest, if you like.

TIP: *This can be close to a pudding, so feel free to adjust the texture to be as thick or thin as you like by using less or more coconut milk. If you do want an actual pudding, add a tablespoon of grass-fed gelatin to the blender and let it sit for a bit or just use less liquid or a fuller-fat coconut milk.*

PB & J SMOOTHIE

INTRODUCING THE COMFORT FOOD SMOOTHIE: a grown-up peanut butter and jelly sandwich—without the bread, and in a glass. Packed with protein to keep you satiated, it is grounding and filling with a balance of sweet and nutty tastes. Using frozen banana might feel good if you have a summertime baby snuggled on hot skin. Just notice if the colder smoothie that results makes you feel chilled and adjust accordingly.

Serves 3

5 tablespoons (75 g) peanut butter

1 fresh or frozen banana, peeled

1 cup (150 g) fresh or frozen berries or ¼ cup (60 g) all-natural fruit jam (no artificial sweeteners, just fruit)

1 tablespoon flaxseed meal (optional)

2 cups (480 ml) light coconut milk or nut milk of your choice

1 tablespoon honey

Blend everything in a blender until smooth. For an extra-pretty presentation, take a knife and smear some of the fruit on the inside of the serving glasses in an upward spiral. Pour the smoothie into the glasses for a striped look that any kids in the house will love.

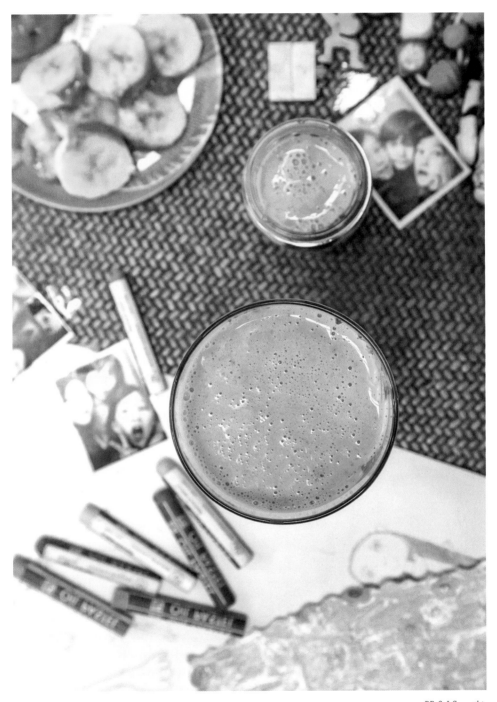

PB & J Smoothie

JOYFUL GREEN SMOOTHIE

WHEN MOTHERS GET THIS SMOOTHIE in their cache of MotherBees meals, they go absolutely gaga for it (an appropriate response given the little one at their side!). It's a smoothie that's as hearty as a soup and its combo of magic plant ingredients has become our special sauce—so addictive I always guzzle the leftovers from the blender pitcher. Adjust the type of greens depending on your digestion, as kale can cause gas if you're not used to it. Parsley adds a fresh, grassy flavor, but for those unaccustomed to green smoothies, it might be too strong a taste to start with.

Serves 2–3

1–2 handfuls of kale leaves or spinach leaves (baby kale is delicious if you can find it)

2 cups (480 ml) coconut water

1 tablespoon almond or sunflower seed butter or peanut butter

½ of a fresh or frozen banana

¼ cup (9 g) parsley leaves

1 tablespoon black sesame seeds

1 tablespoon maca powder (optional)

1 tablespoon spirulina powder (optional)

½ teaspoon bee pollen (optional)

Strip the kale leaves from the stems (not necessary if using baby kale), and discard the stems. Blend all the ingredients in a blender until well combined. Drink immediately.

TIP: *The optional tonic powders will add the crowning touch: malty maca helps stabilize hormones and provide energy while bee pollen infuses you with folic acid and B vitamins—it's an energy tonic in traditional Chinese medicine. Start with tiny doses and see how your body likes it.*

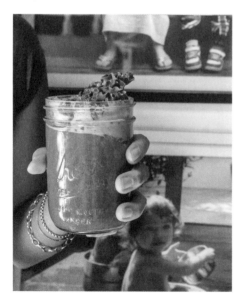

Joyful Green Smoothie

THE FATIGUE FACTOR

While pregnant, you likely fielded many dread-inducing warnings about the sleep deprivation to come, but nothing can truly prepare you for the mind-numbing effects of a sleepless life. Sleep—or the lack of it—is also a huge conversation point for new parents—note how quickly people inquire into your new baby's sleep habits. And note how intrigued you are about the sleep patterns of other people's babies (and note the envy that washes over you when you learn that some infants sleep more than three hours in a row).

If you find yourself patching together a piecemeal semblance of slumber, you're not alone. It's biology, really. Newborn babes need to eat between eight and twelve times a day and usually sleep in three- to four-hour blocks. This makes sense for their tiny digestive systems, but it goes against pretty much everything your body knows about getting a restful night's sleep.

The human sleep cycle is comprised of several phases. The initial non-REM (NREM, or non-Rapid Eye Movement) phases occur when you fall asleep, enter light sleep, and move into deep sleep—which is when the body recuperates physically and the immune system is strengthened. The last phase of the cycle is REM sleep. This is when you process all the data your brain gathered during the day and have intense dreams. It takes about ninety minutes to move into REM. If you are awakened at any stage of the sleep cycle you will have to start the whole process again, and may miss out on the essential REM phase. Sleep is an enigmatic area of study, but research has shown that REM helps us integrate the information we learn; it helps keep our declarative memory—that's the storage of fact-based info like how many ounces are in a cup or the number of states in the United States—running smoothly. REM also influences procedural memory, or the knowledge of *how* to do things. If you don't get enough REM sleep, your body will drop into it quicker each time you fall asleep until you have caught up.

If you pulled all-nighters in college or struggle with insomnia, you may be familiar with the jittery hum of deep fatigue, but it probably never felt quite like this. Baby's cries alone are a jarring alarm clock—one without a snooze button—but you're also feeling the energetic output of breastfeeding and the hormone imbalances that can interrupt the sleep you *do* get. You may be experiencing red and burning eyes; fuzzy brain; cravings for sweet, salty, and fatty foods; chills; grouchiness; or melancholy.

What to do? The baby books tell you to sleep when baby sleeps, but if you have trouble napping during the day you may find it difficult to power down as soon as your little one starts snoozing. A sleeping baby also means that you finally have two hands free to do other things—like wash your face or put on a clean(er) pair of sweatpants. Resist the temptation to tidy the house.

It is absolutely normal to feel tired during these first weeks with baby, but extreme fatigue can be—and should be—avoided. Locking down that crew of support people in your third trimester will help you grab necessary rest whenever possible during the first forty days. Ideally this network of friends and family will pitch in during the early weeks with baby—when your body is in deep recovery mode and solid sleep is especially of the essence. If a neighbor can take your older child to school and if a friend can do a couple loads of laundry, you will be able to maximize possible sleep time. At the very least you will not overload your already taxed system with more to-dos. This is the time to delegate and receive, delegate and receive. Fortunately the uncomfortable effects of sleep deprivation will begin to subside with the addition of just an hour or more of sleep to your daily quota.

snacks

As mother to a newborn, you'll be doing more things with one hand than you ever imagined. That also includes eating. Sometimes you need a quick pop of food that needs no plate or spoon to get you through to the next warm meal with minimal work. These snacks help you fill the gaps without resorting to pretzels, chips, or other processed foods that can feel fun to eat in the moment, but don't fuel your system with sustenance.

You can make a big container of granola during the Gathering—it feels and smells so homey—or if someone asks, "What can I do?" ask them to fill a tin with it, or make a box of healthy crackers. Snacks are gifts that are fun to make and never go wasted. Plus, you'll have something to offer the loved ones that you do let in the door!

You'll also find ideas for super-simple pairings of warming foods that will deliver satisfaction and nourishment in single bites. So while one hand takes care of baby, the other hand keeps you fed.

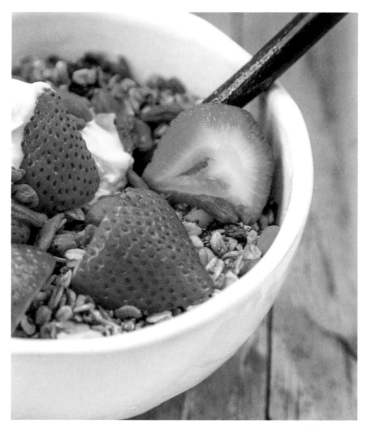

Coconut & Fig Granola

COCONUT & FIG GRANOLA

MAKING GRANOLA IS A VERY maternal and homey project. You get to don an apron, open the pantry, and get hands-on with rustic-feeling foods. I love this version's mixture of spice and sweet and its satisfying contrast of textures. Eat it straight from the jar or toss it in a mug with some milk, nut milk, or yogurt. After baby comes, you'll be happy that the fig seeds are natural laxatives and the nourishing oats are packed with fiber.

Makes 6–8 cups

6 cups (540 g) rolled oats

½ cup (about 90 g) leftover already cooked grains, such as wild rice, millet, quinoa, or buckwheat (optional; see Tip)

1 cup (85 g) shredded unsweetened coconut

1½ cups (225 g) roughly chopped dried figs

½ cup (120 ml) honey or coconut nectar, brown rice syrup, or maple syrup (but not a solid sweetener, it needs to be liquid)

¾ cup (1½ sticks/170 g) salted grass-fed butter or coconut oil, plus extra for greasing the pans

Zest of 1 medium organic orange

1 teaspoon sea salt

1 teaspoon ground cinnamon

1 tablespoon pure vanilla extract

Preheat the oven to 300°F (150°C). Grease two large rimmed baking sheets (or you can line them with parchment, whichever is easier).

In a large bowl, mix the oats, leftover grains, if using, shredded coconut, and figs.

In a medium saucepan over medium heat, slowly melt the honey and butter, stirring frequently. Remove from heat and whisk in the orange zest, salt, cinnamon, and vanilla. Add to the oat mixture, stirring until everything is evenly coated. Spread out on the prepared baking sheets.

Place one baking sheet on the top oven rack and the other on the bottom rack. Bake about 30 minutes, rotating the baking sheets halfway through (from top to bottom) to ensure even baking, and stir frequently, pulling the edges into the middle and pushing the middle to the edges so the edges don't burn. The granola is done when toasted and nicely golden brown in color.

Place the baking sheets on wire racks and let the granola cool. Eat immediately, or store in an airtight container at room temperature for up to 2 weeks.

TIP: *The addition of cooked grains is optional but highly recommended—a great way to use up leftovers and add some unique texture and protein to your granola.*

PEANUT BUTTER, BLACK SESAME, COCONUT & CHOCOLATE GRANOLA

THE GOURMAND'S GRANOLA, THIS ONE is decadent *and* healthy at once, and manages to fold in an Eastern secret of the sages—black sesame. It stores well for weeks, so don't be shy, make a big batch. This granola is a great antidote to a sudden snack craving, with just the right amount of honey to healthfully scratch that need-a-hit-of-sugar itch.

Makes 5 cups

½ cup (120 ml) coconut oil or salted grass-fed butter, plus extra for the pans

4 cups (360 g) rolled oats

½ cup (60 g) chopped nuts of your choice

¼ cup (30 g) black sesame seeds

¼ cup (20 g) shredded unsweetened coconut

2 cups (480 g) peanut butter or almond or sunflower seed butter (or you could use a mix)

1 teaspoon sea salt (if using unsalted nut butter)

¼ cup (60 ml) honey, or more to taste

½ cup (50 g) cacao powder or unsweetened cocoa

1 teaspoon pure vanilla extract

1 teaspoon ground cinnamon

½ teaspoon ground allspice or nutmeg (optional but delicious)

½ cup (85 g) chocolate chips or chunks (optional)

Preheat the oven to 300°F (150°C). Grease two large rimmed baking sheets (or you can line them with parchment, whichever is easier).

In a small pan over low heat, melt the coconut oil until liquid.

Meanwhile, in a large bowl, mix the oats, nuts, sesame seeds, shredded coconut, peanut butter, salt, if using, honey, cacao powder, vanilla, cinnamon, and allspice, if using. Add the melted coconut oil and stir until everything is evenly coated. Spread out on the prepared baking sheets.

Place one baking sheet on the top oven rack and the other on the bottom rack. Bake about 30 minutes, stirring every 10 minutes, pulling the edges into the middle so they don't burn, and rotating the baking sheets halfway through (from top to bottom) to ensure even baking. The granola is done when toasted and nicely golden brown in color.

Place the pans on wire racks and let the granola cool for 8 to 10 minutes. Stir in the chocolate chips, if using. Store in an airtight container at room temperature for about 2 weeks.

CHEESY CRACKERS

SALTY, TASTY, AND ADDICTIVE TO
the max: Homemade crackers are
where it's at when you crave grazing
food. These crackers can easily be
made with gluten-free flour, and will
take different kinds of cheese. They
are not too crunchy, a quality that
would be unacceptable according to
traditional postpartum protocols. Kid
friendly, they do well with dips and
toppings, and they give you something
to serve when a friend drops by for a
tea and a chat—as long as she puts the
kettle on for both of you!

Makes a full 16" x 12" baking pan

1 block cheddar cheese (about 8 ounces/
    225 g), cut into several large chunks

½ cup (1 stick/115 g) salted grass-fed or
    organic butter

1½ cups (190 g) all-purpose flour (or garbanzo
    bean flour for even more protein)

1 teaspoon sea salt, for sprinkling (optional)

Preheat the oven to 375°F (190°C).

In a food processor, mix all of the
ingredients together until you get coarse
crumbs. Slowly pour in ½ to 1 cup (120 to
240 ml) water, pulsing the dough until it hits
the sweet spot when it turns into a large,
fairly smooth ball.

Transfer the dough to a bowl, cover
with a clean kitchen towel, and chill in the
refrigerator for 1 hour.

Roll out the chilled dough directly on
a baking sheet until it's as thin and even
as possible without breaking. For thicker
and softer crackers, roll the dough out a bit
thicker. As you make these again and again,
which I'm sure you will, you can play around
with what you and your family like.

With a sharp knife, score the dough
into squares or rectangles, sized to however
large or small you want your crackers to be.
Sprinkle the sea salt over the top, if you
like, and bake for 20 minutes, or until crisp
and golden. Let them cool on the sheet for
10 minutes and then rescore/slice if needed
to separate the crackers.

Store in an airtight container at room
temperature for 1 to 2 weeks.

THE END OF YOUR ROPE

If you're anything like the millions of mothers who've walked this path before you, parenting will remind you—again and again—that you are utterly and completely human. Your offspring has the power to induce in you the greatest expression of love *and* the deepest well of frustration. You may be wondering how it is possible to be filled with great, nearly overwhelming surges of adoration one moment and pushed to tears of exasperation the next? Welcome to motherhood!

Even the most angelic of babes will push your buttons at some point. This is a standard part of parenting, but unfortunately it's not always expected. The media has been bombarding you with fabricated images of the postpartum experience for as long as you can remember. You know the scene: A smiling, well-rested woman gently sings a lullaby to the softly cooing baby nestled in her arms. Both mother and child are beaming and beautiful. The feeling in the room is sweet and peaceful, like all is right in the world. Does this look anything like the scene in your home, where you've been wearing the same spit-up encrusted yoga pants—the only pants that will fit—for the past three days? Where your laundry is cascading in lopsided dunes across your bedroom floor? Where the piercing sounds that escape from baby ravage your frazzled nerve endings on an hourly basis?

The early weeks with baby can be a wild roller-coaster ride as you negotiate the volatile combination of sleep deprivation, a partner who likely feels neglected, and a demanding little person who won't stop screaming until he gets what he wants (the baby, not the partner—hopefully). Just like adults, no two babies are alike. Yours may be easygoing—eating, pooping, and sleeping like a champ. Or she may not. Babies are often challenging. Their relentless demands, odd schedules, and incommunicative nature make them inherently taxing. If yours happens to be colicky or a light sleeper or a squirrelly nurser (all common newborn traits), your mothering stamina will need to stretch to new lengths.

There will come a moment, one of many, many such moments, where you will feel like you can't take it anymore. You'll feel too tired, too hungry, too overwhelmed. Your baby may refuse to take the nap you've been waiting for since 3 A.M. or she may refuse to nurse when you know she's hungry or maybe she just. won't. stop. crying. The emotions you feel during these moments—severe frustration, anger, sadness, hopelessness—are indicators that you are at the end of your rope. Though rarely discussed, end-of-the-rope moments are an absolutely normal part of parenting. They are not a sign that you're a bad mother or that you're weak or incapable. And they definitely do not reflect upon the love you feel for your baby. End-of-the-rope moments happen to every mother. Nobody escapes. The circumstances will differ, but the feeling will be the same: *I can't take it anymore.*

Experienced postpartum doulas want their clients to become increasingly comfortable with the concept of reaching the end of their rope. Just like you can expect to feel tired during the first forty days with baby and joyful during the early days, you can also count on emotionally jarring moments. During these times, you may find yourself thinking some pretty negative thoughts about being a mother, about your baby, about life in general. It's common to feel ashamed about the thoughts and feelings that come up—mothers are often striving to meet unrealistically high standards of parenting. We're expected to handle more than we've ever handled before and do it with a smile. But just because you gave birth doesn't mean you stopped being a thinking, feeling, emotional being. Mothers are imbued with an array of superpowers, but we aren't robots. Emotions etch a strong line through the postpartum experience, one that will be with you throughout your experience as a parent. Postpartum doulas, the ones on the front lines with new mothers, advise their clients to use their end-of-the-rope emotions as signposts. When you reach the end of your rope, it's a signal that now is the time to turn some energy and love back to yourself—you need a break. With your crack support team in place, you will be able to turn to someone and say, "I need help."

Remember, we used to raise our babies in community. We were enveloped in a group of loving, capable people who would help ease the strain of parenting. Now, isolated from our extended families, we're often doing it alone. But we don't have to. When you find yourself face-to-face with the end-of-the-rope—and you *will*—send an SOS to one of your support people. A simple phone call or text that says, "I really need a break," will have a magical effect. The relief may come in a deceptively simple form: a ten-minute shower, a twenty-minute foot rub, a thirty-minute nap. You may just need someone to hold the baby while you talk for a few minutes or you may need someone to give you a hug and place a hot cup of soup in your hands.

Soon you will see that reaching a breaking point and asking for help to move through it is a natural, expected aspect of motherhood. Your baby will pee, poop, burp, and cry. The sun will rise and set. You will feel joy, bliss, sadness, and frustration. It's all real. It's all okay. Your job is to set down any and all critiques of yourself and simply bring in extra help when things get hard.

CREATE A NEW HABIT: REACH OUT WHEN YOU'RE AT THE END OF YOUR ROPE

If you are prone to beating yourself up when you feel overwhelmed—or too isolated—use the opportunity that is the first forty days to create a new habit. Tell yourself—even write it on a piece of paper and tape it to your bathroom mirror: *When I reach the end of my rope, I'm going to ask for help, love, and attention to come my way until I can figure it out.*

There is always someone who can help. Don't try to muscle through these feelings on your own! There are support hotlines available to help you twenty-four hours a day.

Every mother is going to have times when she's done, when she needs a break.
It's in those times when you feel empty or triggered that you need to be able to call on help,
yet there's a belief in our culture that asking for help is a failure. I work with
mothers to normalize the need for help.

—LINDSAY GERMAIN, POSTPARTUM DOULA, SAN FRANCISCO BAY AREA, CA

BLUEBERRY & OAT PANCAKES

These fun-to-make snacks are staples in my household, where three kids always need extra energy to carry them through until lunchtime. They also provide tasty sustenance for the new moms whom I serve. The nutrients from steel-cut oats are absorbed into the blood more slowly than regular oats, which delivers energy in a sustained manner. They're also an exciting treat for those following a wheat-free diet, who may have been longing for a plate of pancakes but never knew to try making them with oats!

Serves 6–8

1 cup (160 g) steel-cut oats

1 pinch of sea salt

4 tablespoons salted grass-fed butter or coconut oil, plus more for serving

¼ cup (60 ml) milk of your choice

1 teaspoon pure vanilla extract

1 tablespoon olive or avocado oil

½ cup (120 ml) yogurt or kefir

2 large pasture-raised eggs

¾ cup (95 g) gluten-free flour, plus more if needed (chickpeas or almond flour optional)

½ teaspoon baking powder

1 cup (155 g) frozen or fresh blueberries

1 banana, peeled, quartered, then sliced

1 tablespoon chia seeds, finely chopped walnuts, or hemp seeds (optional for added crunch)

Maple syrup, honey, or cooked fruits for serving (optional)

In a small pot, combine the steel-cut oats with 2 cups (480 ml) water and the salt. Bring to a gentle boil over medium-high heat, then reduce heat to low, give it a gentle stir, and cook, three-quarters covered, for 20 minutes or until tender. Remove from heat and add 2 tablespoons of the butter. Set aside.

In a large bowl, whisk the milk, vanilla, and olive oil with the yogurt, and then add the eggs and whisk until incorporated. Stir in the flour and baking powder, and then add the blueberries, bananas, and chia seeds, if using. Add the oat mixture to the batter and stir to combine. The consistency should be thicker rather than runny. If you need to add more flour, you can do that now.

Melt the remaining 2 tablespoons butter in a nonstick pan over medium heat. When the pan is nice and hot, scoop or spoon the batter into the pan, making either one large pancake per batch, or two or three small pancakes at a time if the pan will hold them. Cook over medium heat for 3 to 4 minutes on each side, flipping to the second side when the batter bubbles on top. Transfer the pancakes to a plate when golden on both sides. (The cooking times tend to speed up the more the pan heats up, so keep a careful watch.) Add more butter to the pan for each batch.

Serve the pancakes warm with butter, and if you like, maple syrup or honey. Or keep them in the fridge for a snack whenever you like. You can heat them up in a toaster oven very quickly; they're delicious topped with almond or peanut butter, too. They also freeze well if you can't eat them all up in a few days.

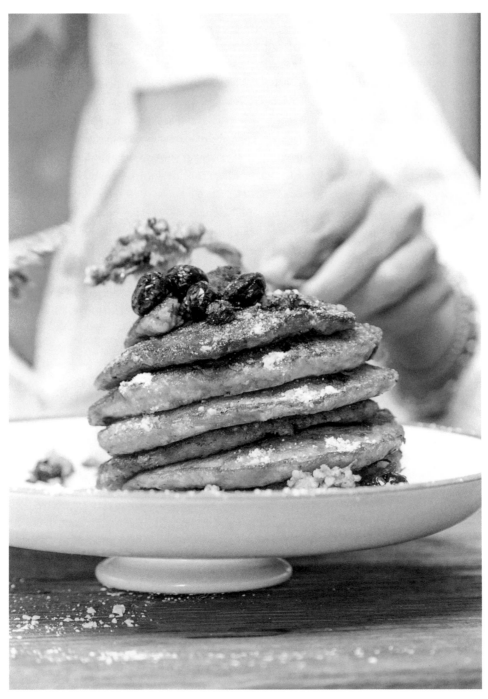

Blueberry & Oat Pancakes

sweets

Mothers deserve to be celebrated! Gorgeous, curvy, loving, tender, and strong—a woman with her child is a beauty to behold. But sometimes in the shuffle of diapers, the reality is that she feels anything but. These delectable desserts are offered as a reminder of your sensual side. Dip your spoon into a luscious egg custard; let your tongue linger on a bite of soft chocolate mousse. Sink your teeth into a coconut confection. These low-sugar treats are a reminder that life is sweet. They use raw honey—one of nature's sexiest foods, and considered a panacea in Eastern medicine—or coconut sugar, both of which should be enjoyed in moderation but do include important minerals and other micronutrients as a benefit.

"Sweet" is a taste that is actually used in healing arts, to ground you when overly airy or anxious, and to help moisten the inner body. These quick treats take the place of way-too-cold ice cream or over-sugared candy and they make magic out of things you already have in your pantry. You can enjoy them knowing they're packed full of ingredients that bring health benefits alongside the pleasure.

If it feels like the sexy woman you were before is lost forever in a sea of sweatpants and ponytail holders, take five minutes and treat yourself. She'll be back. She never really left—she's just busy right now. And meanwhile, there's chocolate.

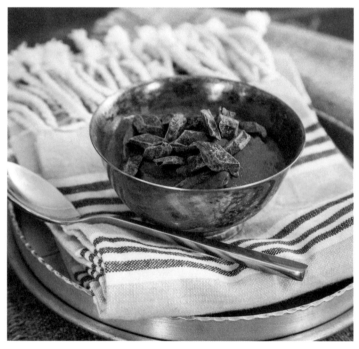

Chocolate Mousse

CHOCOLATE MOUSSE

DECADENT AND CREAMY, YOU'D NEVER know the main ingredient in this sinful-seeming dessert is your friend the avocado! I love to stash this in a mother's fridge so she can enjoy a few spoonfuls when she needs a sensual treat. You have full license to eat it however you please—with a blob of almond butter, with shredded coconut and fresh berries, or heaped onto a base of leftover granola in a ramekin, like a mini chocolate-cream pie.

Serves 6–8

2 ripe avocados

¼ cup (60 ml) raw honey, coconut sugar, or maple syrup

½ cup (50 g) cacao or cocoa powder (you could also use carob powder or some combination)

1 tablespoon coconut oil

1 tablespoon pure vanilla extract

½ teaspoon sea salt

¼ cup (60 ml) water or nut or coconut milk of your choice (as needed for thinning to desired consistency)

¼ cup (60 g) almond or peanut butter (optional)

1 teaspoon unflavored gelatin, preferably Great Lakes grass-fed brand (optional)

Optional toppings: crushed nuts, cacao nibs or chocolate chips, shredded coconut, dried fruit like mulberries or sliced Turkish figs, goji berries, bee pollen

In a food processor or blender, mix the avocados, honey, cacao, coconut oil, vanilla, and salt with ¼ cup (60 ml) water (or choice of nut milk or coconut milk) until smooth and creamy. If the mousse seems too thick, add more water or milk, a little at a time, as you don't want to make it too thin.

Serve with whatever toppings you want. Store leftovers (if any!) in an airtight container in the fridge for several days.

TIP: *Although optional, the gelatin adds extra nutrition and a custard-like texture.*

VANILLA COCONUT HAYSTACKS

PILLOWY AND LOVELY, COCONUT HAYSTACKS are as sensual and luscious as your curvy, mother's body. They are soft and yielding—the food equivalent of a contented sigh—and because they're full of protein from the egg whites and healthy fat from the coconut, you get well fed while you revel in their bliss. For an extra and unique fragrance and heart-opening element, add a few drops of rose water to these treats; it's a perfect pairing with the vanilla.

Makes 1 dozen

6 large egg whites (save the yolks for custard or mayo)

½ teaspoon sea salt

½ cup (120 ml) honey

2 tablespoons pure vanilla extract

4½ cups (385 g) shredded unsweetened coconut

2 or 3 drops rose water (optional)

Preheat the oven to 350°F (175°C). Grease a baking sheet with coconut oil or butter.

In a medium bowl, whisk together the egg whites and salt until stiff peaks form. Gently mix in the honey, vanilla, shredded coconut, and rose water, if using, until just combined. Don't overmix or you'll deflate the egg whites.

Drop tablespoons of the batter onto the greased baking sheet, pulling the tops up a bit when you lift the spoon away to form a tiny, rounded mountain peak (like a chocolate kiss) each time.

Bake for 8 minutes and check. If the haystacks are not turning slightly golden yet, leave them in the oven for another 4 minutes. Most likely total bake time will be 10 to 12 minutes. Remove the haystacks from the oven when they're just a bit golden on the outside and still soft inside.

Let cool on the pan or on a wire rack for 3 to 5 minutes. Serve warm or room temperature.

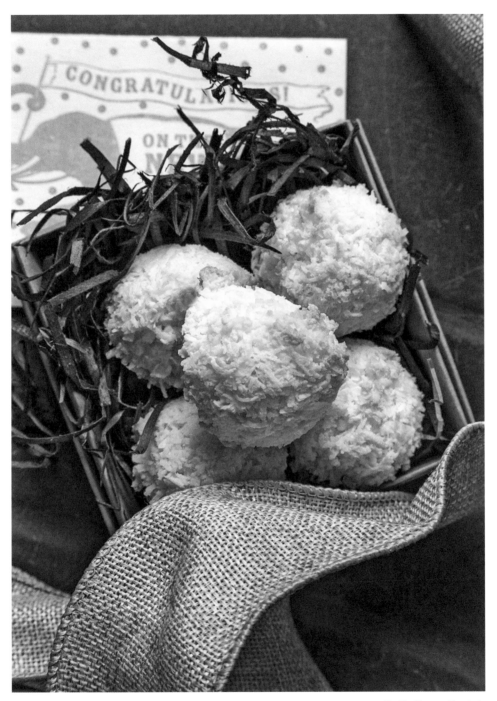

Vanilla Coconut Haystacks

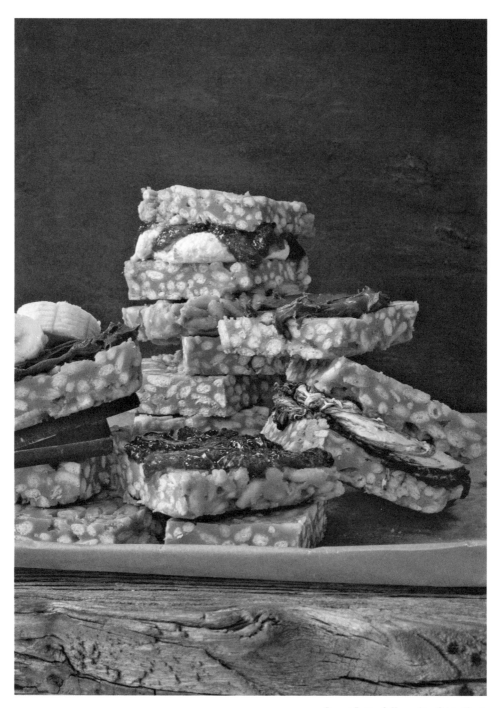

Peanut Butter & Honey Rice Crispy Treats

PEANUT BUTTER & HONEY RICE CRISPY TREATS

NOTHING MAKES YOU GROW UP quickly like becoming a parent. These treats permit you to feel like a kid again. They are a snap to make and the peanut butter is so much better than the marshmallows found in packaged versions. (Almond or sunflower seed butter are fine substitutions.) Goji berries, raisins, or crunchy-sweet fig pieces work great as add-ins.

Makes an 8-inch square pan

1 cup (240 g) peanut butter

½ cup (1 stick/115 g) salted grass-fed butter

½ cup (120 ml) honey

2 cups (30 g) organic puffed rice

Pinch of sea salt

Optional add-ins: chocolate chips, peanuts, shredded coconut, dried fruit of your choice

In a small saucepan, melt the peanut butter, butter, and honey over medium heat, stirring until well combined.

Put the puffed rice in a mixing bowl with the pinch of sea salt, add the peanut butter mixture, and stir until the cereal is evenly coated. Stir in any optional ingredients you'd like. Transfer the mixture to an 8-inch (20-cm) square pan and press down gently to cover the bottom. Chill in the fridge for at least 20 minutes, or up to several hours. When they are hard to the touch, cut into squares and enjoy. They will soften at room temperature, so best to keep them chilled until you are ready to eat.

SPICED VANILLA EGG CUSTARD

CUSTARD IS ICE CREAM BEFORE it's frozen—a sumptuous blend of egg yolks and cream that melts in your mouth. This super-simple version uses coconut milk and a very pure and nutrient-dense powdered gelatin to help it set. Go wild, because with the yolks, coconut, and gelatin, it's perfect postpartum nutrition! Experiment with add-ins and toppings. You can even serve it in little ramekins with burnt sugar on top.

Serves 6–8

1 teaspoon unflavored gelatin (I use Great Lakes grass-fed gelatin)

2 cups (480 ml) full-fat coconut milk from a carton

¼ cup (50 g) coconut sugar or ¼ cup (85 g) honey

1 teaspoon pure vanilla extract

1 teaspoon ground cinnamon

1 teaspoon ground allspice or ½ teaspoon ground nutmeg or cloves

4 large egg yolks

Place 1 tablespoon water in a small bowl, stir in the gelatin, and set aside.

In a medium saucepan, combine the coconut milk, sugar, vanilla, cinnamon, and allspice.

Bring to a gentle simmer over medium-low heat and continue simmering for about 5 minutes, stirring occasionally to make sure the milk doesn't scald or stick to the bottom of the pan. Meanwhile, whisk the egg yolks in a medium bowl. After 5 minutes, gradually add ½ cup (120 ml) of the coconut milk mixture to the egg yolks, whisking briskly for a minute or two.

Reduce heat to low and whisk the egg yolk mixture into the remaining cream mixture in the pan. Continue to whisk constantly, until the custard is thick enough to coat a wooden spoon, about 5 minutes. Add the gelatin and whisk or stir until dissolved. Remove from heat and divide among six to eight small ramekins or the cups of a muffin tin. There isn't a set amount for each serving; make them as large or small as you like.

Transfer the custards to the refrigerator (sometimes putting them on a baking sheet makes this easier, if you have the space in your fridge), and chill until set, at least 4 hours. If not serving right away, cover the custards with plastic wrap and chill for several days.

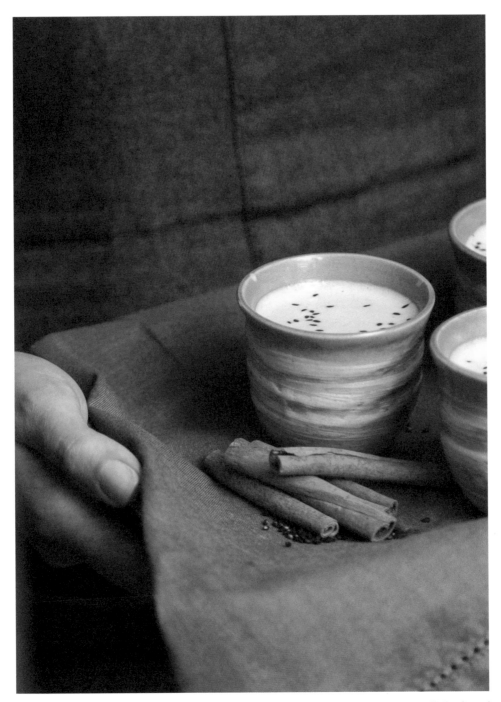

Spiced Vanilla Egg Custard

TO MOVE OR NOT TO MOVE?

"Workout" and "weight loss" are not in the first forty days vocabulary. This tender window of time is not the moment to "get back" in shape or "bounce back" to your pre-pregnancy body—no matter what supermarket tabloids say about svelte celebrity mamas (who are hopefully not hitting the gym in this phase anyway)! It is a time to take a conservative approach and overestimate your need for recovery. Most doctors and midwives advise no exercising save for gentle walks before the six-week mark, and certainly no heavy lifting as the uterus finds its way back to a nonpregnant position. Traditionally, the new mother would be "confined" to the home so she couldn't get any wild ideas about jumping about outside.

If you're an athletic or outdoorsy person, you might balk at the idea of limiting your movements. But your body might have the final say: Many women find that even walking too much, too soon, can exacerbate bleeding. Let the postpartum discharge complete almost entirely before you wander afield, so that your body's "gates" can close. Should you choose to go out in these weeks, wrap baby snugly on your chest in a baby carrier, keep your own body warm and protected, too (remember those Indian ladies wearing woolens in the summertime!), and make your strolls short.

Often, what we're craving from exercise is the elevation of mood we know it will deliver. I love to share two simple, heart-opening body postures with new mothers that have instant mood-enhancing effects (and that can be done right next to baby's bassinet). Heart-opening poses make you feel better because they expand the throat, chest, and lower-back areas, helping to stimulate the release of energizing hormones while mitigating stress-response hormones.

The victory pose is a yogic power pose that mimics the euphoric celebratory posture of a runner crossing a finish line. Stand tall with feet planted hip-width apart, hands on hips, chest expanded open. Now lift your arms over your head into a V for "Victory," let your back arch slightly, look up at the sky, and smile! Research shows that two minutes of this raises energy-giving testosterone by 25 percent and reduces stress-inducing cortisol by 15 percent, while helping to build confidence and self-esteem. Try a few twenty-second stints of this posture throughout the day at first, building up to longer if you like.

A restorative heart-opener pose is priceless for those moments when even standing up feels like a stretch. Place your exercise ball against the wall and sit on the floor with your back against it. (Crossing your legs may be helpful here.) Lean back and rest your head on the top of the ball and let your arms fall softly open on each side. Relax into the ball and feel your chest plate open and your neck get longer. Close your eyes and breathe in through the nose and out through the mouth. Hold for as long as you like. This one posture alone can bring sweet relief to body and spirit: It lets you nurture yourself by doing (literally) nothing at all.

TIP: *If you don't own an exercise ball, fold a thick bath towel in quarters, then roll it into a tube, place on the floor, and lie down with your spine along it and your head just coming off the end of it onto the floor. Relax as above, with arms and knees falling open.*

GOOEY CHOCOLATE BROWNIES

THESE GLUTEN- AND DAIRY-FREE BROWNIES are decadently healthy treats, rich and chocolaty. Plus, they are big on healthy fats and protein, which balances out and slows down possible blood sugar spikes. Kids and adults will adore them—be prepared to share the recipe!

Makes 12 large brownies or up to 24 bite-size brownies, depending on how they're cut and how strong your chocolate cravings are!

¾ cup (70 g) cacao powder or organic cocoa powder

1 cup (125 g) gluten-free flour of your choice (or leftover nut pulp from straining homemade nut milk; see pages 182-183)

¾ cup (175 ml) honey, maple syrup, or coconut nectar

1 cup (240 g) almond butter, peanut butter, or cashew butter

2 large pasture-raised eggs

¾ cup (180 ml) almond milk or nut milk of your choice

2 teaspoons vanilla extract

1 teaspoon baking soda

½ teaspoon sea salt

6 ounces (170 g) dark chocolate bar of your choice

¾ cup (130 g) dark chocolate chips or chunks for extra chocolate flavor (optional)

½ cup (45 g) shredded coconut or walnuts (optional)

Preheat the oven to 325°F (165°C). Grease a 13 x 9-inch (33 x 23-cm) baking pan with coconut oil.

Put the cacao in a large bowl then add the next 8 ingredients, mixing well and slowly to avoid a cloud of cacao powder poofing up into your face, as has happened to me before!

In a small pot over medium-low heat, slowly melt the 6 ounces of dark chocolate, stirring frequently, being careful not to burn it. Remove from heat when it is just barely melted.

Add the melted chocolate to the bowl along with any optional ingredients you choose and stir a few times until just incorporated, leaving some streaks/swirls in the batter if you like. Pour the batter into the prepared baking pan and spread out evenly. A wooden spoon or spatula helps here.

Bake the brownies, setting a timer to go off after 15 minutes. Rotate the pan 180 degrees, reset the timer for another 15 minutes, and bake. The brownies are done when the edges are firm, but the insides are still gooey and melty. If they are still extremely gooey in the center, bake for a few more minutes, taking care not to burn the outsides. (If they do end up too dark for your liking, simply trim the outside edges off with a knife.)

Let the brownies cool in the pan for at least 10 minutes before slicing them and removing them from the pan, otherwise they'll fall apart. (Though I must admit I almost never let them sit that long without sampling some!)

hot drinks

The kettle has a starring role in traditional **zuo yuezi**, because teas are integral to the postpartum protocol. The new mom sips hot or warm drinks all day the way many of us in the West swig cool water. It's not simply for hydration, which is super-important in the postpartum period. Tea is also the first and most obvious way to bring heat to your insides; hot water settles the "wind" that can get into the now-vacant baby room—your womb—and that can then whip through the whole house of your body to cause discomfort and distress. Then, of course, there are the ingredients steeped in the water that are chosen for their therapeutic effects.

The wise women who traditionally surrounded a woman during pregnancy, birth, and over the days and weeks that followed knew that Mother Nature has special gifts to offer the childbearing woman. Her leaves, fruits, roots, flowers, and weeds can be used to relax or rebuild a new mother's depleted body, to help her breasts lactate, and to settle the mind or even to energize her when fatigued. These natural wonders are the ultimate folk medicine—cheap to source and safe to use.

During the first forty days, reframe the cup of tea from a once-a-day beverage to an all-day affair. Let warm tea be your companion from dawn to dusk (and through to dawn again). Or let it cool to room temperature and sip it from a canteen instead of plain water. You may be surprised that these natural remedies include everyday things such as oats or nettles. But these are our overlooked allies in taking good care of ourselves as women.

Gathering supplies of herbs, sorting and storing them in mason jars, and brewing them with boiling water is such an ancient and feminine art. It is an earthy ritual that will move you with its mystery—the wisps of aromatic steam and the sensations in your stomach, or breasts, or mind—even if you are the most urbane type of woman. As you practice tuning in to how your body responds to different brews, you don't just get the benefits of, say, greater lactation or sweeter sleep. You are developing that intuition, that listening within, that will be your greatest tool as a mother.

TEAS & INFUSIONS

Steeping herbs in hot water is the simplest way to experience the healing power of herbs. When a small amount of an herb is steeped for just a few minutes to extract the plant's beneficial oils, it is a tea, with mild but palpable therapeutic effects. When a large amount is steeped for several hours, it becomes an infusion, more potent and more medicinal in effect. You'll enjoy these teas' harmonious flavors, and may find infusions to be more intense. Herbalists say that infusing herbs unlocks the minerals, vitamins, and even proteins in the leaves for deeper nourishment of the whole body.

NETTLE & FENNEL TEA

TOTEMS OF SPRINGTIME AND NEW life, nettles energize the body with a satisfyingly textured, creamy taste, and support the liver, helping to detoxify any impurities like pharmaceutical or anaesthesia drugs in your system. Fennel is another classic childbearing herb; it has estrogenic properties that can help hormone balance, boost lactation, and ease digestive upset in baby or mom. For all those reasons, this blend is a first forty days staple.

Serves 6

1 cup (27 g) dried nettle leaves
¼ cup (about 25 g) dried fennel seeds

Bring 6 cups (1.4 L) water to a boil in a medium pot. Add the nettle leaves and fennel seeds, lower heat, and simmer for 30 minutes to an hour, covered.

Strain and drink warm or store in the fridge for up to 3 days.

VARIATION: Add 1 cup (200 g) uncooked barley to the fennel and nettle water at boiling point, then add an extra cup of water (240 ml), lower heat, and let everything simmer over low heat, covered, for 30 minutes, until barley is softened. If it gets too thick, add more boiling water, ½ cup (120 ml) at a time.

RED DATE & GOJI TEA

THE QUINTESSENTIAL *zuo yuezi* TEA with its wonder-duo of warming ingredients, this is a daily must-drink for all moms, in my opinion, and a big flask of it can sit by your side all day. It is sweet and tart, and its crimson-colored fruits remind you to tend to your expanding, emotional heart.

Serves 4–6

2 cups (about 160 g) red dates (see "Pantry Resources," page 124)
½ cup (55 g) goji berries
Your choice of sweetener, such as honey, maple syrup, coconut sugar (granules or syrup), or stevia to taste (optional)

Bring 6 cups (1.4 L) water to a boil in a medium pot. Halve the red dates and add them to the boiling water. Reduce the heat to a simmer and cook for 1 hour, covered. In the last 20 minutes, add the goji berries and your desired sweetener. (The red dates provide enough sweetener for my taste, so I normally leave it out.)

Strain and sip throughout the day, or store in the fridge for up to 1 week.

INFUSIONS

The following six herbal infusions are time-honored postpartum herbs, in slightly new combinations for a twist of flavor. Many of these herbs are powerful galactagogues—lactation enhancers.
To prepare: Place the dried herb and other ingredients in a 1-quart (960 ml) mason jar; fill with 4 cups (960 ml) boiling water and cap tightly. Strain after 4 to 8 hours.

TIP: *I recommend making these infusions before you go to bed so they're ready the next morning. Refrigerate what you don't drink or drink within the day, hot or at room temperature.*

NETTLE INFUSION

IMPROVES MILK FLOW AND QUALITY, and is rich in iron and protein. This one gives a tingle of energy that feels almost euphoric. If it's springtime and nettles are available at the farmer's market, you can make a fresh version. It's great during your third trimester to nourish you and throughout postpartum, too.

1 cup (22 g) dried nettle leaves
2 lemon slices (add when you are about to drink)

RASPBERRY LEAF INFUSION

IMPROVES UTERUS STRENGTH BOTH BEFORE and after birth, enhances milk flow and quality. Raspberry leaf is a nice-tasting herb that is a classic pregnancy tonic. Drink during the third trimester and after the birth.

1 cup (15 g) dried raspberry leaves
2 cinnamon sticks

RED CLOVER INFUSION

THIS HERB IS A LACTATION enhancer and blood nourisher; also a classic liver-support tonic, which is great for hormonal balance. It's slightly strong-tasting and a good substitute for black tea if you are hankering for a cup. The lemon tempers the flavor.

1 cup (14 g) dried red clover blossoms
1 lemon slice (add when you are about to drink)

GOAT'S RUE INFUSION

THIS LACTATION ENHANCER HAS A slightly grassy, earthy taste. Fennel gives an extra layer of flavor and additional lactation-enhancing effects.

1 cup (40 g) dried goat's rue
¼ cup (70 g) fennel seeds

BLESSED THISTLE INFUSION

A LACTATION ENHANCER THAT PROVIDES emotional support and alleviates depression. Fenugreek is a classic lactation-boosting spice.

1 cup (28 g) dried blessed thistle

¼ cup (36 g) fenugreek seeds

MOTHERWORT INFUSION

IDEAL FOR CRAMPING AFTER BIRTH or any traumatic feelings from the birth experience. Also, relieves uterus pain and lifts depression. Use this herb lightly if there is heavy bleeding. Do *not* use while pregnant.

1 cup (28 g) dried motherwort

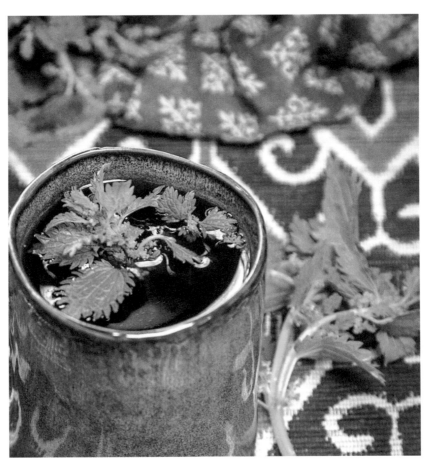

Nettle Infusion

GINGER, TURMERIC & HONEY TEA

TURMERIC IS A WONDER FOOD. It's a rhizome (root) with superb anti-inflammatory and antibacterial effects that pairs beautifully with honey and ginger. This tea is a tonic for the whole body after the efforts of childbirth. Add some heated coconut milk for a thicker, creamier drink.

Serves 4

1-inch (2.5-cm) knob of fresh ginger, peeled and grated (about 3 tablespoons)

1-inch (2.5-cm) knob of fresh turmeric, peeled and grated (about 3 tablespoons)

2 tablespoons apple cider vinegar

¼ cup (60 ml) honey, or to taste

Bring 5 cups (1.2 L) water to a boil in a medium pot. Turn off heat, add the ginger, turmeric, and vinegar. Let it steep, covered, for 10 minutes.

When you are ready to drink, stir in the honey. Leftovers keep in the fridge for up to 1 week.

TIP: *You can purchase fresh turmeric in Asian groceries and some natural foods stores, but if you cannot find it, a teaspoon of powdered turmeric can be used instead.*

FINDING BALANCE IN THE BUSYNESS

Though the complex juggling act that is modern motherhood is a significant part of life, contemporary society does not have adequate structure in place to support women who work and have children. If you are one of the millions of women who will very soon be balancing professional responsibilities with caring for your children, your relationship, and your household, meeting the numerous demands of your very full life will require a special kind of attention to your own needs. As the pace picks up, it will be essential to keep up your nutrition and hydration (this is doubly important if you are still nursing), recognize when you are fatigued, and turn to your loved ones when you need to vent, cry, or laugh. These are not expendable, optional action items. They are necessary steps to keeping you fortified and capable of delivering all that is being requested of you. As you foray out into the world, keep your self-care supplies with you. You can whip up a Joyful Green Smoothie and take it on the road in an insulated bottle. The same goes for Chicken, Red Dates, and Ginger Soup, Nettle and Fennel Tea, or any type of congee, which goes easily to the office in a lightweight metal container known as a tiffin. You can take ninety seconds to allow a hard emotion to move through you, or you can rub a few drops of a soothing essential oil on the inside of your wrists or the palms of your hands—lavender works wonders for stress and anxiety—and breathe the scent in deeply.

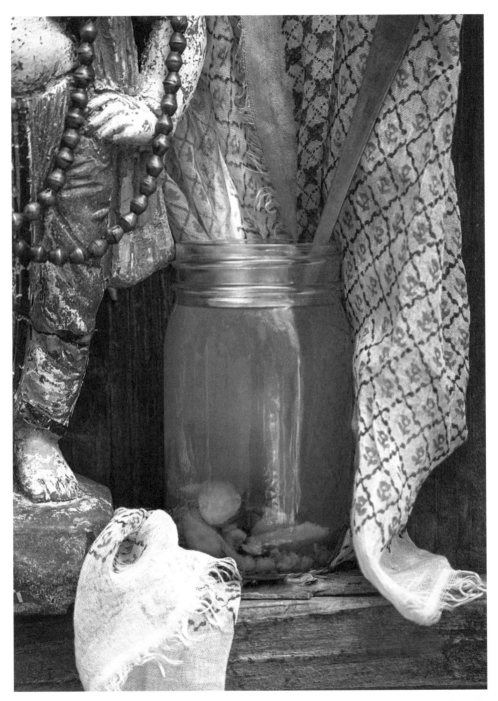

Ginger, Turmeric & Honey Tea

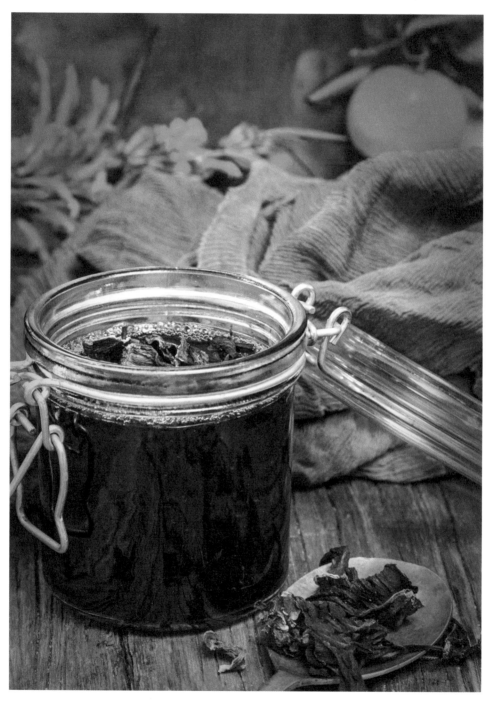

Hibiscus Flower, Ginger & Cinnamon Tea

OATS, GINGER & CINNAMON TEA

REMINISCENT OF MEXICAN *HORCHATA*, THIS BEVERAGE IS circulation-boosting, warming, and rich with the lactation-supporting benefits of oats.

Serves 4

1 cup (90 g) rolled oats

½ cup (40 g) steel-cut oats

1½-inch (4-cm) knob of fresh ginger, peeled and halved

3 cinnamon sticks or 2 tablespoons ground cinnamon, plus more ground cinnamon for sprinkling

Pinch of sea salt

1 to 2 tablespoons honey, or to taste

Bring 7 cups (1.7 L) water to a boil in a medium pot. Add the oats, ginger, cinnamon sticks, and salt to the boiling water. Reduce heat to low and let it simmer, three-quarters covered, for 30 minutes. Check to make sure the water level remains the same, adding more water if needed. Keep an eye on the pot, as it is very easy for this tea to boil over.

When the water has turned a milky white color and the mixture has a smooth consistency, strain it, saving the oats for another use (congee or cookies come to mind!). Pour the tea into a glass jar or directly into your mug, then stir in the honey. Sprinkle the top with a touch of ground cinnamon and drink warm.

Store in the fridge for up to 3 days. Reheat by adding a little boiling water, stir, and enjoy!

HIBISCUS FLOWER, GINGER & CINNAMON TEA

SWEET, FLORAL, AND SPICY, THIS fragrant, warming tea has a wonderfully feminine feel. It is delicious served hot or at room temperature.

Serves 4

4 cinnamon sticks

1 cup (35 g) hibiscus blossoms

1-inch (2.5-cm) knob of fresh ginger, peeled

4 to 5 tablespoons (60 to 75 ml) honey or organic agave nectar (optional)

Bring 4 cups (960 ml) water to a boil in a small pot, along with the cinnamon sticks.

Reduce heat to low, add the hibiscus blossoms, and simmer for 30 minutes, covered.

Turn off heat, grate the fresh ginger into the pot, and let it all steep for 20 minutes. Strain and sweeten as desired and sip throughout the day.

CUMIN & FENUGREEK TEA

A PAIRING OF TWO QUITE everyday spices known to aid lactation and calm the digestion, this slightly bitter-tasting tea is a refreshing counterpoint to the sweeter teas in your repertoire. It can be sipped before nursing.

Serves 4

½ cup (145 g) cumin seeds or ¼ cup (25 g) ground cumin

½ cup (145 g) fenugreek seeds

1 tablespoon honey or coconut sugar, or to taste (optional)

Bring 4 cups (960 ml) water to a boil in a small pot. Turn off heat, add the cumin and fenugreek, and let steep, covered, for 2 to 4 hours.

Strain and sweeten as desired and sip throughout the day.

TIP: *Go easy on the sweetener: This tea is a digestive aid and its bitter taste really gets the digestive juices flowing.*

GOAT'S RUE & OATSTRAW TEA

A SLIGHTLY MORE ADVENTUROUS LACTATION-BOOSTING tea that may involve some specialty herb purchasing online, goat's rue improves milk flow and quality and oatstraw is superb for calming the mood. The taste is quite grassy and earthy.

Serves 4

½ cup (20 g) goat's rue

½ cup (10 g) oatstraw

1 tablespoon honey or coconut sugar, or to taste (optional)

Bring 4 cups (960 ml) water to boil in a small pot. Turn off heat, add the goat's rue and oatstraw and let steep, covered, for 2 to 4 hours.

Strain and sweeten as desired and sip throughout the day.

DELUXE DRINKS

These two steamy drinks are creamy, sweet, and deeply satisfying. Mix them up when craving a luscious treat or when in need of some comfort in a cup. Each drink can be as sweet as you like—some days may call for a spoonful of sugar (preferably raw, and if possible, organic) or a hearty dollop of honey.

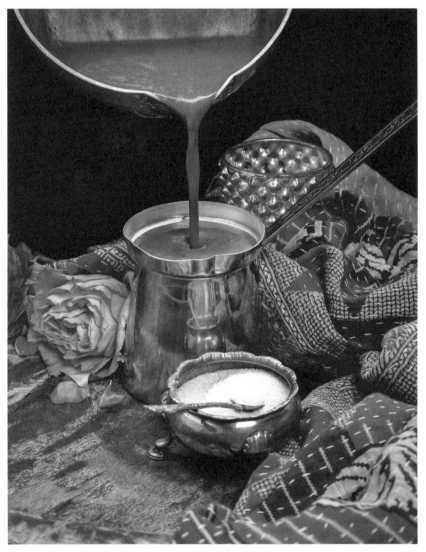

Ceremonial Hot Chocolate

SLEEP NECTAR

THIS SOOTHING AND SETTLING WARM drink is what I prescribe when a mother has trouble relaxing into rest. Warm milk of your choice, plus honey, chamomile, and lavender will help to calm the nerves and tell the body it's time to sleep.

Serves 2

2 cups (480 ml) milk of choice

2 tablespoons chamomile blossoms

2 tablespoons lavender (optional)

1 tablespoon honey

In a small pot, bring the milk to a gentle boil. Add the blossoms and lavender, if using, to the pot (or directly to mugs with the hot milk), cover, and steep for 4 to 5 minutes. Stir in the honey and reflect on your day, feeling blessed.

CEREMONIAL HOT CHOCOLATE

THIS ABSOLUTELY GORGEOUS, MEXICAN-STYLE ELIXIR is inspired by Shell Walker Luttrell, Arizona midwife and creator of the breastmilk-sharing resource Eats on Feets. She goes into the kitchen of every mother she assists right after birth and quietly creates a hot cacao and cornmeal concoction. Can you imagine any better celebration of mom's powerful act? The addition of cornmeal to this drink gives it some substance, and with belly filled, mom can turn her full attention to the amazing being she has just birthed. Drink this during the first forty days—or anytime—and feel free to blend it for a smoother consistency, as the cornmeal does add some texture, which I personally love.

Serves 2

2 cups (480 ml) light coconut milk or almond milk

3 tablespoons cacao powder or unsweetened dark cocoa powder (you could also use carob powder here)

Pinch of sea salt

½ teaspoon chili powder

1 tablespoon coarse cornmeal

1 tablespoon coconut oil, ghee, or salted grass-fed butter

1 teaspoon ground cinnamon

Honey, maple syrup, or coconut sugar to taste (optional)

1 small strip of orange peel (optional)

In a medium saucepan over medium heat, warm the coconut milk, and then stir the rest of the ingredients into the milk slowly.

When the cacao and sweetener are dissolved and it tastes perfect to you, drink warm. There may be some congealed bits of cornmeal, which add lovely texture, but you also can blend the drink until it's smooth if you prefer.

body products

The food you eat is only one aspect of being nurtured and nourished. It's also so much about the touch you receive from others and the kindness you give to every part of yourself. With a vulnerable newborn needing constant care, it's all too easy for your body to feel like a fueling station and for your mental self to run the show.

These nonedible recipes help restore the balance, inviting you to stay in touch with yourself through small rituals of self-care each day. Using basic ingredients from your pantry, they will lavish your body, mind, and senses, or help heal tender skin. As you take twenty minutes to sit in a sitz bath, take the time to thank your body. As you rub oil across your belly, let your moving hands honor the power of your womb.

Making these body products is a lovely project to do with friends, perhaps as part of a gathering before or after baby is born. Then let one of those loved ones bathe, scrub, and anoint your feet—and maybe paint your toenails, why not? Being touched and tended to by others is a mother's birthright, and awakens the part of her that feels beautiful, and precious—two of the most healing and "happifying" energies she can feel.

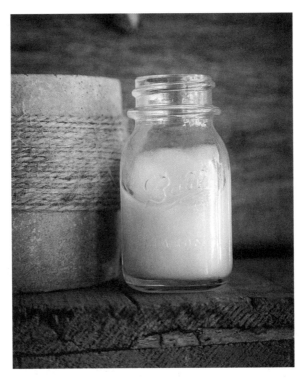

Rose & Coconut Body Oil

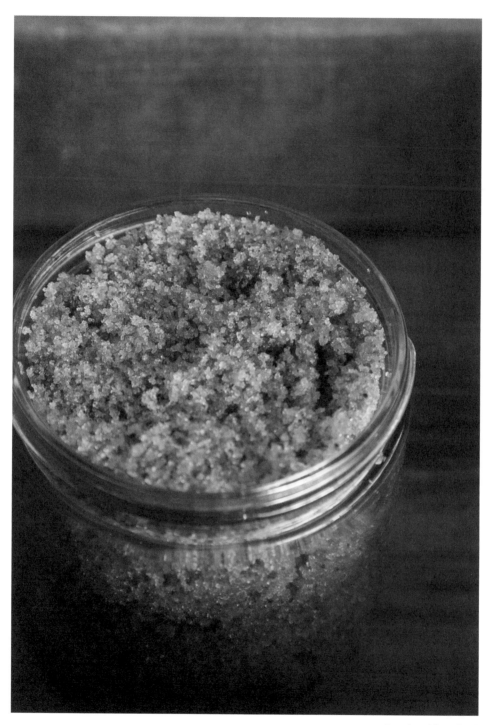

Gingerbread Sugar Scrub

GINGERBREAD SUGAR SCRUB

COMBINE MOUTHWATERING SPICES FROM YOUR pantry to create a wintry, sugary, and gingery cookie-like scrub. Used in the shower, it makes your skin feel luxuriously exfoliated, cleansed, and moisturized—but it's gentle enough for a glow-producing face treatment as well. I like to use it as a foot scrub, as part of a deluxe foot rub ritual for mom. I'd like to imagine every mom receiving this sweet ritual from a friend or her partner. There's no need for reflexology skills; even an amateur foot rub can stimulate the entire body, helping to energize what's lagging and relax what's tense.

Makes about 2½ cups (600 ml)

1 packed cup (220 g) brown sugar

1 cup (220 g) raw cane or turbinado sugar or even coconut sugar (any sugar more coarse than brown sugar)

½ cup (120 ml) avocado oil (or other good carrier oil, such as almond or jojoba)

½ cup (120 ml) melted coconut oil (see Tip, next page)

1 tablespoon pure vanilla extract

1 tablespoon ground ginger

1 teaspoon ground cinnamon

1 teaspoon ground allspice

1 teaspoon ground clove

½ teaspoon ground nutmeg

Mix all the ingredients in a large bowl until well combined. Transfer to wide-mouth mason jars with lids.

Use liberally in the shower or on the face and lips no more than three times a week (no need to exfoliate every day). Keep the jars sealed so it doesn't dry out.

ROSE & COCONUT BODY OIL

Massaging your whole body with warmed oils before bathing is a caring ritual you can do for yourself whether you have two minutes or twenty. Saturating the skin with natural oils feels incredible and, on a deeper level, it calms the nervous system; the oil soothes the aggravating wind that is stirred up inside by the action of birth and can cause anxiety and unease. In India, this daily self-massage is called *abhyanga* and involves rubbing oils like coconut or sesame in long strokes over every part of your body, front and back, using circular motions on the joints, and, if you like, on the scalp as well. The effect is soothing and grounding. (Tradition recommends that you do this while standing on a bath mat, in a warm room, and letting the oil sink in for ten minutes before showering or bathing.)

Using natural oils more simply as a pre- or post-bathing moisturizer will work its magic on your body and senses as well. This coconut oil blend, infused with the scent of roses from inexpensive culinary rose water, is my favorite thing to leave in a mother's bathroom. It encourages her to slow down and take just a few minutes for herself, while someone else tends to baby. Rose is an aroma that awakens the heart—make sure to put your hands on that area, and tune into what your heart has to say.

Makes about ¾ cup (180 ml)

3 tablespoons refined coconut oil
½ cup (120 ml) almond or jojoba oil
1 tablespoon food-grade rose water (available at kitchen supply stores or online)

If the coconut oil is solid, melt it very slowly over low heat, watching carefully so it doesn't smoke or get too hot.

In a small clean jar with a lid, mix the liquid coconut oil, almond oil, and rose water. It will be fragrant with the smell of roses and coconut. Seal the jar and keep it on hand to use often!

TIP: *Coconut oil tends to be liquid in the hot summer months and solid at cooler temperatures. To help keep it more liquid in colder weather, keep a jar of coconut oil near a warm heat source (or in a bathroom where steamy showers are being taken).*

COMFREY SITZ BATH

MOST MIDWIVES AND MANY
OBSTETRICIANS will talk to you about
sitz baths—a remedy for soothing the
tender area around the perineum that
involves sitting in shallow, warm water
infused with skin-soothing herbs.
You can purchase ready-made blends
of herbs, but it's very easy to make
your own. Comfrey and calendula
are renowned for their skin-healing
properties and lavender soothes.
You can use this "body infusion"
blend in three ways: as a sitz bath, for
making frozen maxi pads to reduce
swelling, and to fill a peri bottle to
gently cleanse the entire area between
the legs, especially after going to the
bathroom.

Makes enough for 8 frozen maxi pads

½ cup (15 g) comfrey leaves
½ cup (18 g) dried lavender
½ cup (5 g) calendula blossoms
8 overnight maxi pads (optional)

In a medium pot, bring 6 cups (1.4 L) water
to a boil. Add the comfrey, lavender, and
calendula, remove from heat, and let steep for
20 minutes, covered.

Strain the tea water, then use it in a sitz
bath, transfer to a peri bottle, or dip the maxi
pads into the tea, one by one. Twist each pad
gently to wring out the excess, then place
them, one next to the other, on a baking sheet
and put the pan in the freezer. When the pads
are frozen, stack them in a zip-tight plastic
bag and return them to the freezer until after
your delivery. To reduce swelling in the first
two to three days after birth, you can sit on a
frozen pad for 7 to 10 minutes at a time.

TIP: *For high-quality comfrey, lavender, and
calendula, look no further than Mountain Rose
Herbs (mountainroseherbs.com). This online
retailer sells certified-organic teas, herbs, and
spices that are perfect for pampering yourself
during the postpartum period and beyond.*

afterword: beyond the first forty days

As the first forty days come to a close, you may be feeling like yourself again—or, more accurately, the next version of you. You have fulfilled the silent agreement you made with yourself upon embarking on this period of dedicated rest and rejuvenation. You have given yourself what generations of women have had before you—a stopgap, a period of integration and adaptation, between one chapter of your life and the next.

The time you spent tucked in bed, the good food you fed yourself, and the space you created to adjust to this new life with baby has likely paid off. Good work! During this time, you navigated unfamiliar ground, learning how to breastfeed—or figuring out what to substitute if necessary—and how to soothe and rock and change your little one. Things that were once terrifying and foreign are a lot more familiar now. You discovered reserves of patience and compassion that you didn't know you possessed and tapped into the endless depths of a bright and clear maternal love. Along the way, you may have bumped up against frustration, loneliness, confusion, or sadness. Face-to-face with the great paradox of the postpartum period, you probably felt some or all of these emotions in the course of one day—or one hour.

Now you may be ready to look up from the cooing bundle in your arms and turn your gaze outward. If the first forty days was your chrysalis, your safe space to get messy and transform, you are now ready to emerge as something new, to stretch your wings and show the world the mother you have become. As this unique season of your life comes to an end, keep in mind that forty is a loose guideline, not a hard deadline or a finish line that must be crossed. Forty days, or about six weeks, is the general time frame within which new mothers begin to notice that they are feeling stronger, more energized and more capable and confident in caring for their babies. But you may find that fifty or sixty days is your magic number, or that you are ready to move into the larger world at day thirty-five. There is no right time to move beyond the postpartum period, only the time that is right for you.

As you embark on all that's awaiting you beyond the first forty days, you should find that you are well prepared to move forward. The things that you learned in the past six weeks—how to ask for help; how to cook a steaming, delicious pot of soup; how to honor your body (and your mind and heart, too); and tend to your relationship—will accompany you throughout your life as a parent. While all of the recipes, rituals, and tips in this book are designed to support